HOMOEOPATHY
FOR TEENAGERS

GW00384050

By the same author:-

Homoeopathic Medicine

The Homoeopathic Treatment of Emotional Illness

A Woman's Guide to Homoeopathy

Understanding Homoeopathy

Talking About Homoeopathy

An Encyclopedia of Homoeopathy

The Principles, Art and Practice of Homoeopathy

Emotional Health

Personal Growth and Creativity

The Side-Effects Book

HOMOEOPATHY FOR TEENAGERS

A Guide to Remedies for the Adolescent Years

by

Dr Trevor Smith
MA, MB, BChir, DPM, MFHom

INSIGHT

Insight Editions
Worthing, Sussex
England

WARNING

The contents of this volume are for general interest only and individual persons should always consult their medical adviser about a particular problem or before stopping or changing an existing treatment.

Insight Editions
Worthing
Sussex
England

Published by Insight Editions 1994

© Trevor Smith 1994

Trevor Smith asserts the moral right to
be identified as the author of this work.

British Library Cataloguing in Publication Data

A catalogue record for this book is available
from the British Library.

ISBN 0-496670 16-1

Cover photograph by the author.

INTRODUCTION

The adolescent years are an extension of childhood and a recapitulation of many childhood needs - for example there is a constant need to have something in the mouth. In early childhood it was a dummy or thumb, in adolescence it is usually a cigarette, sweet, pen, or a drink. There is enormous preoccupation with appearance, large portions of the day given to self-examination and care, particularly of the skin and hair, which take on an enhanced sexual symbolic significance.

The teenage years are particularly difficult, because at the same time as dependency needs on both parents, there is a strong drive to move away from them. Each teenager needs to establish his own identity. This is an oscillating process, which is often very painful for the young adolescent, and often for the family. It can cause a combination of childish needs, as well as provocative, aggressive, unreasonable behaviour, which at times seems insensitive and out of character.

The teenager repeats all the demands of the young child, within his adolescent frame, but fired this time by the libidinal motor. Rapid growth occurs from about the age of twelve, beginning earlier in the girl, shortly afterwards in the boy. There is a pressing need for warmth, comfort, food, acceptance, recognition and above all reassurance.

At the same time, childhood needs are still present within the rapidly growing adolescent body, often re-emerging as childish insecurities, selfish behaviour and immature personality demands to test-out and challenge.

All of these pressures and needs create difficulties in relationships, particularly towards adults and authority.

The male teenager feels uncomfortable within his changing body envelope and is concerned with issues such as strength, virility and body hair. The girl is usually waiting for her first period to arrive, or coping with often painful, irregular, heavy periods for the first few years. Adolescents tend to feel that they are the only ones experiencing these sorts of problems, isolated and ashamed of their body and emotions, reluctant to discuss or express their sense of vulnerability. There are frequent problems communicating with anyone outside their immediate peer group, mainly because it is a time of such intensity - with fluctuating moods, ideas and ideals, everything carried to extremes.

Adolescence is also a time of need for support, especially for psychological reassurance. The typical adolescent feels awkward and vulnerable, as he struggles to put on a brave face of youthful experience, competence, suavity and well-versed accomplishments, including knowledge of the risks and pitfalls of sexuality. He asserts this competence to relate to others, in spite of feeling painfully trapped in a psychological no-mans-land, neither child nor adult, shy and insecure, alternatively aggressive, noisy or violent. Every teenager needs a great deal of time and understanding by his family and should be helped to realise that his parents have gone through similar problems and come through them. The adolescent finds great relief when he understands that his parents can appreciate his problems and understand from their own experience what he is going through because of the hormonal, metabolic, physical and psychological adjustments he must make.

Adolescence is not a time for great decisions about life, although ideals are often established and kept throughout the adult years. Provided the adolescent stays in touch with himself as an individual, with fears and difficulties, he will be in a better position to understand himself. Later he may also be more able to help his own children when they have adolescent problems. Parents should always be available and 'on call', to discuss areas of interest, concern or difficulty and especially when the teenager needs clarification and help.

When childhood has been satisfactory, with a good relationship between the parents, open communication, discussion of problems and anxieties, the teenager is more likely to go into puberty with reasonable confidence.

Parents can help teenagers by using a natural approach (such as homoeopathy), for physical and psychological problems, because it harmonises with each adolescent stage of formation without imposing or creating additional pressures. Homoeopathy does not cause side-effects which undermine health. The remedies used will not throw the delicate adolescent balance into chaos at a time when the physiological and psychological systems are changing and easily harmed by anything which is not in tune with biological responses.

A healthy childhood, with problems treated in a sensitive way, as they arise, makes for a more healthy adolescence.

Some psychological stress inevitably occurs in childhood, including bullying, physical abuse, separation, hospitalisation, surgery, problems within a one-parent or step-family, bereavement, loss of a parent, sickness or illness of one or both parents. One patient, seen recently, had parents with a schizophrenic illness. This frequently required admission to hospital because of confused or violent behaviour. The inevitable instability at home created severe social problems for the adolescent who felt shy and guilty, ashamed of his parents and angry because he could not invite his friends back to the family home.

Where problems can be dealt with in a healthy way by discussion, anxieties are less likely to occur in adolescence. This open healthy approach is recommended whenever homoeopathy is used.It is also found that where problems are talked through at the time of a trauma, often in childhood, they do not re-emerge in such an intense overwhelming way during the adolescent years because they have already been given the attention needed.

Adolescence is always a time of turmoil, psychological upheaval and uncertainty, because the most profound aspects of the person are re-experienced at this time. Homoeopathy is of value because it helps put much of this emotional turmoil into balance. It also makes it easier for adolescents to accept the feelings and reactions which emerge. In this way they do not feel so strange, unusual, or alienated. This is one of the most important roles of homoeopathy for this age-group.

Every age and stage of growth is important, but it is particularly important to treat the adolescent as a person, respect, value and listen to his viewpoint. Even the most difficult and challenging awkward teenager must be listened to, his opinions recognized, and his world seen through adolescent eyes.

Parents must learn to appreciate the adolescent's viewpoint even if they don't agree with it. The opinions although immature or extreme, nevertheless have an appeal and a freshness to them, an idealism, which the parents lost many years ago. What the adolescent feels so strongly often causes upset because it reminds the parents of their own early lost ideals, hopes and standards.

Few adolescents are able to carry such high ideals into adult life and bring them to fruition, which is a common cause of later adult depression, frustration and dissatisfaction.

Parents should learn from these contacts and discussions. It can also help them to re-think their own attitudes and priorities.

The most difficult area for parents is adolescent sexuality because of the surging power of the youthful libidinal dynamo. This is usually on the surface of the teenager at a time when parental libido is declining. The mother may be on the pill, her libido low, the father tired or exhausted so that his sexual drive has diminished. As a result, adolescent drive and libido can be felt as a threat, leading to resentment, jealousy and attempts by the parents to limit or downgrade enthusiasm and drive. A mother can feel jealous or threatened by a teenage daughter. A father may become jealous of his son. Such intense feelings on both sides, easily slip into point-scoring, pain, hurt and conflict.

No adolescent should become a threat to parents however insecure. He should be a source of pride and satisfaction, an extension of his childhood and a life which they have contributed to. The healthy parental role is not to hold down adolescence but to acknowledge and give it support, help to bring it to maturity, showing the options and opportunities available and how adolescent drive can be used for positive purposes.

In this way adolescent energy can be channelled into a wide variety of artistic and social interests, sport and creative expressions. Only when the flow of adolescent drive and energy is blocked, is there a danger of it becoming diverted into drugs, smoking, alcohol, crime and violence.

Adolescents should be encouraged to talk - not just at school, but in the home - about their feelings and sexual problems. Parents should also talk more about their own experiences and problems at this time and how they set about solving them. These areas should be treated as normal and not be avoided, as if in some way they are unnatural. Teenagers should also be encouraged to talk about any areas which concern and worry them - particularly sexuality and money.

It is still unusual for mothers to talk to their daughter about her periods, or for fathers to discuss the significance of a 'wet dream', what it signifies and how it relates to healthy normal masculine development.

Such powerful emotional areas are too often shut down and avoided, left for teenagers to discuss in the playground or club. In this way they become associated with secrecy, shame, or guilt and find an outlet through unhealthy energy drives.

When parents and teenagers are able to be more free and open, to give more information and especially to discuss sexual matters as something essentially healthy and normal - there will be fewer teenager pregnancies and abortions and also less risk from smoking, drugs and AIDS.

7, Upper Harley Street
London NWI 4PS

ADVICE ON TAKING HOMOEOPATHIC REMEDIES

The remedies recommended throughout the book should be purchased directly from a homoeopathic pharmacy or health shop. Always ensure that your remedies are from a reliable source and taken in the 6c potency.

The potencies or strengths, come as small round pills or tablets, made of sucrose (or lactose). If you are sensitive to lactose, you should order your remedies directly from a homoeopathic pharmacy, requesting a sucrose or lactose-free pill base for the remedies. Because the medicine or homoeopathic dilution is applied directly to the surface of the pill, they should not be handled. They are best placed directly into the mouth from the lid of the container, and sucked under the tongue. They should always be taken at least 30 minutes before or after food or drink (except water), orthodox medicines, vitamin or mineral supplements and toothpaste.
Do not drink peppermint tea when taking homoeopathic remedies. Also avoid coffee, tea, and cocoa.

The medicines should be stored in a cool, dry, dark area, away from strong odours, especially camphor, oil of wintergreen, perfume, essential oils, after-shave, and soap. In this way, their action will last indefinitely.
A bland diet is recommended, not eating to excess, or using strong spices. Alcohol should be avoided, and smoking should be reduced or stopped.

Remedies should be taken for as long as any symptoms persist - and then stopped. If new symptoms arise during homoeopathic treatment, they should be watched carefully, especially if they have occurred in the past. The homoeopathic action may sometimes cause earlier symptoms to reappear. They are usually fleeting, but if persistent, they will require a new remedy.

An 'aggravation' of symptoms, after taking the remedies, is a positive sign. It is usually short-lived, and does not undermine the overall sense of well-being. Do not continue taking a remedy once the symptoms have improved.

There are no side-effects or risks from homoeopathy. If you take a wrong remedy, or a whole box of the 6c pills, they will cause no harm. The remedies can be safely used during pregnancy, breast-feeding, or given to the youngest baby.

Homoeopathic remedies do not interact with orthodox medicines, or undermine their action. Some drugs, especially steroids, may reduce or neutralise the homoeopathic effect.

Homoeopathy is not a treatment for acute or severe pain, and orthodox treatment is recommended if this occurs. Homoeopathy acts at every age, the reaction varying with age, strength, and the resistance or vital energy reserves of the patient. It acts very quickly in a child, or fit young person, but is slower in an elderly person, particularly if old, weak, or feeble.

It is often better initially, to give an orthodox treatment to an elderly person during the acute stage of an illness, using homoeopathy when they are recovering, or before they are in acute illness or weakness.

ACNE

The common condition of teenage spots with recurrent often itchy, round and red thickened areas of the skin which may become infected and chronic. It is common on the face, but may also occur on the chest and back or in any greasy area of the skin. The condition is harmless and although the cause is still not clear, it is thought to be related to hormonal changes, or to a diet that is too high in sugars. These create an artificial diabetes in the skin areas allowing bacteria and yeast organisms to flourish. It is a very common teenage problem, and most adolescents have acne at some time. It is particularly distressing because at this age adolescents are preoccupied with their appearance, especially of skin and hair. Any form of spot or blemish may become a source of teasing or shame, embarrassment or awkwardness. Many teenagers 'work' at their acne, rubbing, cleansing and applying endless creams and lotions which aggravate the condition, because they provide a moist environment for bacteria in addition to the high skin sugar levels. Worst of all they often try to pick off their acne spots and scabs which leads to secondary infection, or a chronic condition with risks of future scarring.

The skin should be left alone when acne is present, the affected area kept clean with a cleansing cream rather than with soap which tends to block the pores. Because of the risks of secondary infection, rubbing or endless touching of the skin should be avoided. The diet should contain high quantities of raw fresh vegetables but kept low in refined sugars. Because of the high fructose or fruit sugar content of most fruits, these should also be eaten sensibly and not to excess. Avoid any fruit, for example oranges, that aggravates the condition.

Remedies to consider:

Antimonium crud   For infected acne, the area painful and irritated with swollen dark red areas which discharge pus. All symptoms are worse for heat, especially at night, causing scratching to the point of bleeding.

Graphites   For dry crusty acne which oozes, usually a thin clear or straw-coloured liquid. The discharge may be sticky and is usually worse at night from the heat of the bed.

Petroleum   The area is thickened, red, dry and irritating. The main problem is a tendency for the skin to crack deeply and to become infected.

Pulsatilla   Symptoms are variable,the acne intermittent, worse from a high intake of either sweet or hot foods, such as chocolate, also aggravated by heat or emotion.

Rhus tox   There are thickened, swollen, intensely irritated areas, causing a strong desire to scratch to the point of bleeding.

Sulphur   The skin is irritated, looks grey or unclean, discharging pus.

15

AGORAPHOBIA

Fear of open spaces and places where the teenager feels exposed and under scrutiny or unprotected. This is a common problem of adolescents as well as adults and reflects a loss of security and a fear of going out into unfamiliar or public places, especially where there are other people, queues, or any situation where they might be held up and delayed from getting home. The teenager may feel fine in the near-neighbourhood, within a close area near to home, but panic arises when faced with going outside the circle, or to anywhere new. All security is firmly rooted in the home and family, rather than within the individual and there is a wish to stay home, to avoid school or college, often with physical symptoms of malaise, fainting, lack of energy, weakness, a sense of collapsing which may lead on to a fear of dying. Psychologically the clinging reflects an internal struggle between wishes to be strongly independent and more explorative and adventurous, and a contrasting wish to stay home where it is safe. Frequently strong ambivalent feelings to one of the parents are present. These may have never been openly declared or talked through, becoming something secret, linked to guilt and shame. In the younger teenager, such feelings may become associated with a fear of something happening to a much-needed parent, often the mother, especially if she is not at home all the time. Typical anxieties which occur are that she may become ill, might die, or leave the family home. Such fears are usually rooted in either a family emotional crisis between the parents, with a sibling, or a close member of the family has died or moved away. The teenager agoraphobia often reflects a failure of the family to communicate and function openly as a unit.

Remedies to consider:

Argentum nitricum There are strong phobic problems with fear and insecurity, all symptoms worse from heat, or any new situation.

Gelsemium There is an over-emotional reaction to going out, meeting people, attending school, with lack of confidence, hysterical outbursts, apathy and withdrawal based on fear of contact with others. Lack of competitiveness is a common problem.

Natrum mur Indicated for lack of confidence and fear of others. There has usually been some psychological damage in childhood, which has led to the belief that any form of closeness with others is a threat. He is tearful, often depressed, rigid in attitudes, fearing change of any kind.

Silicea For the teenager who lacks confidence, 'grit' and staying power, too willing to take fright and stay away from any challenging or new situation. He is usually small and thin physically, as well as weak psychologically, but the main problem is lack of confidence.

ALCOHOL

One of the commonest of all teenager outlets from frustrating or stressful situations which he feels cannot be adequately expressed in a more direct or mature way. It is common in both male and female teenagers and usually associated with cigarette smoking. Many teenagers drink in moderation and can control the habit without being excessive, but others use it as a barely concealed social prop for feelings of vulnerability and unhappiness. Drink in itself is not harmful in small amounts, but in excess, alcohol is a cerebral depressant and makes the handling of problematic relationships or emotional situations more difficult than they need be. Because alcohol depresses and inhibits the brain, it also lessens the brakes on violent or risky behaviour, such as drug-experimentation or frequent changes of a sexual partner.

The alcohol habit tends to undermine the health and natural resistance of the body and as it takes hold, leads to neglect, failure to eat a wholesome diet, and severe psychological depression. It is a classical form of escape from being unable to talk about problems within the family or job, dealing with other people of the same and opposite sex, or those who are felt to be in authority. All of these are issues and problems to some degree for every adolescent, but where verbal or social skills are lacking, usually from inexperience, they are even more of a task, and alcohol is often felt to be the only way of easing tension, being less 'up tight' with others, or feeling a failure. The main problem is often that the alcohol habit tends to make any underlying problem far worse and leads to even further alienation from problem-solving and maturation for the teenager.

Remedies to consider:

Avena sat For mild alcoholic problems. The main problems are insomnia, lack of concentration and exhaustion.

Natrum mur Indicated where the drinking is due to underlying depression and lack of confidence. They are usually solitary drinkers who are anxious in the presence of others.

Nux vomica There is a combination of short-fuse emotion and intensity of feelings, often caused by lack of confidence, anger and rage at the success of others and underlying depression. They are often violent with alcohol.

Pulsatilla For variable intermittent drinking, the person often needing company and a boost. The underlying feelings of inadequacy and shyness tend to become worse with alcohol leading to tearfulness and feeling sorry for their plight. All symptoms are aggravated by heat and alcohol.

Silicea Where weakness and lack of confidence is the major problem and alcohol seems the only way to find 'dutch courage' and a temporary source of stamina.

ALLERGY

Hypersensitivity, or severe reaction to specific irritants in food, drinks, drugs or the environment, is now one of the commonest causes of illness and time lost from work or college by adolescents. Desensitization skin tests have usually been tried and failed, the patient often showing a sensitivity reaction to a variety of different substances. Allergy to pollen with chronic nasal catarrh, itchy eyes and a post nasal drip are frequent, also hay-fever from grasses or pollens. Some teenagers suffer from asthma due to hypersensitivity to feathers, various domestic animals, or to house-dust mite, often waking up at night with spasm of the chest and short of breath, usually worse when the weather is hot or humid. Some have a skin allergy to plants, flowers, or sprays, others to eating certain fruits or foods, to colourants in drugs, or convenience foods or drinks. Others are allergic to the oils in woods, such as rosewood.

Many teenagers have a reaction to chlorine after swimming, with conjunctivitis, nasal and throat catarrh. In all of these allergies there are at least two factors at work. One is the emotional health of the adolescent because allergy has been clearly shown to have a psychological element and the reactions can either be brought about or totally inhibited on one side of the body by hypnosis. The other factor, which is of especial interest to the homoeopath, is the underlying health, resistance and vitality of the individual patient. Where this background level of health has been weakened for any reason in the past, it must be improved to increase overall health, as plants must have their soil and root-system improved to increase resistance to disease. See pages 25 and 76 for allergic asthma and hay-fever.

Remedies to consider:

Kali carb   Where there are recurrent allergic problems such as asthma or hay-fever, associated with being over-weight and lack of energy. All symptoms are aggravated in the early hours, often waking with an aggravation in bed at 4-5.00 a.m.

Phosphorus   For the teenager who is popular, out-going and energetic, but with a weak chest and tendency to allergic conditions. He is usually thin and tall, always chilly, yet prefers cold food and drinks.

Sulphur   For the teenager who is overweight, always hot and sweating, lacking will-power, full of ideas which are never put into practice. His general health is poor, picking up every infection that is in the family, sweating, grumbling and usually unhappy, with a poor achievement record. All symptoms are aggravated by contact with water.

Tuberculinum   A miasmic remedy, often indicated to treat inherited allergic traits or areas of weakness.

The constitutional remedy of the teenager may be required, usually prescribed by your doctor.

ANOREXIA NERVOSA

This is a common problem of the adolescent due to profound insecurity problems. It may be acute or sometimes long-term, the body weight dropping as low as four stones (56 lbs) and becoming life-threatening. It is much more common in girls than boys, but may affect either. It often begins with a period of bulimia or compulsive eating, with bingeing on certain foods, such as chocolates or ice-cream or both, followed by obsessional dieting and attempts to lose weight rapidly. The attempts to crash-diet lead to self-induced vomiting and the use of laxatives in a determination to get rid of the 'bad' food they have previously eaten and the discomfort and feelings of being blown-up and distended. Eventually the whole area of eating and food becomes a psychological obsession which dominates every moment of the day and every activity, causing misery and anxiety. As the weight drops, menstruation stops and fat is lost from essential organs including the heart. The stomach shrinks from chronic lack of any substantial food within in, which then causes the most intense discomfort as soon as food is taken. There is a tendency to pick and to pretend to eat more in company, as food is hidden whenever possible. Vomiting leads to pain and discomfort, to tearing of the lips at the corners, to weakness and loss of a normal regular sleep and bowel pattern. The condition is serious and may at times be fatal. Anorexia is not a condition that is suitable for self-treatment and it is essential that it is treated by a doctor. At times hospitalisation may be required. It is important to help the adolescent understand his distorted self-imagery, anxieties about sexuality and any other fears that may be present.

Remedies to consider:

Pulsatilla

There is an underlying lack of confidence, symptoms very changeable and variable, with frequent tearfulness and dramatic emotional outbursts. All symptoms are aggravated by heat and the presence of others because of the need to be at the centre of attention. There is an extreme obsessional preoccupation with the body, appearance and terror of putting on any weight, despite the daily evidence of the dangers of low body weight.

Phosphorus

For the more confident teenager, who is thin, always cold, likes others, is popular, often very talented artistically, but with a distorted body image. There is a tendency to recurrent chest infection and he is always chilly, but paradoxically, at the same time prefers ice-cold drinks.

Tuberculinum

For the thin, chilly, anxious teenager, constantly preoccupied with weight and dieting. Self-induced vomiting is common. The teenager is often depressed and lacks confidence. Most symptoms are worse on waking and during the morning, better for fresh-air.

APPENDICITIS

This is an acute inflammation of the appendix organ of the intestinal tract, near the ileo-caecal valve, or where the small and large intestines join. The appendix is a blind tract or small side cul-de-sac part of the intestine which can easily become infected or blocked.

Often a grumbling appendix is caused by a series of minor infections in the area, characterised by lower abdominal pains, usually on the right side, although where the position of the intestinal organs is reversed, it can occur on the left side. The area is tender and associated with colicky pain, often nausea and sometimes constipation or diarrhoea.

Where the patient is in a collapsed state - the abdomen hard, like a board, obviously ill and weak, usually with a pale white tongue, a slight temperature - then he should be seen by a doctor as soon as possible to ascertain if surgery is required.

Where the attacks are mild - the teenager not really ill, mainly suffering from mild lower abdominal right-sided discomfort, with no raised temperature or vomiting, not off his food - then the condition can be safely treated by homoeopathy. But if in doubt get a medical opinion.

Remedies to consider:

Lycopodium   For recurrent low right-sided pain, usually associated with indigestion and upper abdominal distention. Most symptoms are worse in the late afternoon or early evening, improved by movement, but aggravated by local heat. The symptoms are paradoxically improved from warm drinks.

Nux vomica   The pains are colicky and spasmodic, associated with marked irritability of mood.

Ornithogalum   For recurrent right sided abdominal pain with vomiting, distention and belching. There are also severe upper abdominal pains after eating.

ASTHMA

Asthma is usually associated with tightness or spasm of the bronchial tubes, from a wide variety of causes.

The major symptoms are shortness of breath, with wheezing, high-pitched noisy breathing, and exhaustion. Symptoms are often worse at night, frequently after midnight as the temperature falls, aggravated by effort, as games and sport, also from any psychological stress situation.

Asthma is a common problem of adolescents who have a family history of asthma, or sometimes another related allergic conditions, as hay-fever, migraine, or eczema. In some asthmatics, there is no family link to its causation and attacks occur quite independently of any inherited genetic causes. Asthma is considered a psychosomatic illness, because there is often an emotional causative component to it, although this is not necessarily the major factor causing the breathing difficulties. Wheezing often follows an acute chest infection such as pneumonia, whooping cough, after measles or influenza, which weakens the lung defences and vitality. The onset can also occur after a family emotional crisis, although in many asthmatics there is no obvious cause for the onset.

Asthma is commonly associated with allergy to pet hair, colourants in foods, dairy products, pollens or grasses.

During an attack, the parents should remain calm and reassure the child, keeping him warm and sitting upright. It often helps to moisten the air, using a steam kettle.

26

Remedies to consider:

Kali carb   For recurrent asthmatic problems in an overweight, flabby teenager who lacks energy and confidence. All symptoms are worse in the early hours as the temperature drops, usually from 4-5.00 am.

Medorrhinum   Asthma is usually associated with chronic catarrh and sinus problems. Mouth breathing often occurs, with a post-nasal drip on lying down causing coughing and throat irritation. Chest symptoms are improved from sea air and humidity.

Phosphorus   The teenager is typically thin and pale, flushing-up easily from emotion and over-reacting to the least excitement. He is popular and talented with plenty of energy, but quickly becomes short of breath from effort, a throat infection, or catching a cold. Every infection seems to go to the chest causing wheezing and breathing difficulties. The asthma is worse from hot weather, also from damp cold and thundery conditions. He always feels cool or has cold hands, but prefers cold drinks to warm ones, which tend to aggravate chest problems.

27

ATHLETE'S FOOT

A usually chronic fungal infection, mainly occurring between the toes and common in schools and particularly swimmers. The fungal spores are present on the floor of the baths or changing rooms or on towels.

The condition is encouraged when the area between the toes is not properly dried after swimming or running. It is not a general health risk to the adolescent but is unpleasant and often itchy and painful. In some adolescents it occurs without any link to sport and is caused by a tendency of the feet to perspire.

The condition may sometimes become more severe and chronic, and involve the whole of one or both feet, also the hands with a painful irritating rash, which cracks and bleeds, making walking or running uncomfortable.

Regular salt water baths are helpful, also bathing the feet in a weak solution of Potassium Permanganate, using a few drops of 1% solution.It is important to dry between and under the toes. Wiping between the toes with an alcohol solution after drying helps to prevent fungal infection. Pool slip-on shoes, should be worn in the changing area, shower and when walking to the edge of the pool.

Remedies to consider:

Arsenicum iod   For itchy dry or scaly areas of the foot, in a teenager who is often tired and exhausted with a poor circulation. The feet are always cold, often damp with sweat. Other symptoms which indicate this remedy are recurrent fevers and a rapid pulse.

Calendula   The remedy supports healing of fungal infections. All symptoms are worse for cold or damp weather.

Sepia   The toes are often damp from perspiration, all symptoms worse for water application, cold, thundery conditions. Moods of irritability and exhaustion are worse in the evening.

Thuja   The feet sweat profusely, the skin olive-coloured and oily. Warts tend to recur, especially on the feet. The condition is worse at night from the heat of the bed, typically, about 3.00am.

BAD BREATH

This is a distressing problem for many adolescents when they particularly feel vulnerable, unattractive or unlovable, reinforcing any insecurity they feel about themselves. The most common causes are dental, either due to caries and infection or there is a food trap between a filling which if not flossed daily leads to its content putrefying which is clearly sensed in the breath.

Other causes are a chronic sinus or throat infection, indigestion - usually from eating too quickly and the wrong foods which ferment in the stomach. The main dietary error, is to take foods which are rich in sugars, especially sweets or chocolate snacks, or any quickly satisfying convenience type of food. Smoking and alcohol are other important causes. The problem usually disappears as the general health and diet improves and any dental problems and food traps are corrected.

Always ensure that the adolescent has a daily bowel movement to help elimination, and to prevent the accumulation of stagnating gassy digesting food. This is best achieved by giving a high-fibre food in his diet, ideally a balanced breakfast cereal. This should contain bran and be sugar free. A daily salad made with fresh raw vegetables will also help cleanse the body and improve the problem. Parents should ensure also that the teenager eats raw fruit as part of his everyday diet.

Remedies to consider:

Carbo veg   A very useful remedy where there is upper abdominal flatulence with distention. Fermentation and gassy formation is common, most symptoms worse from eating rich foods, in the evening or heat.

Kali bich   The bad breath is associated with sinusitis, the throat or nose constantly blocked. All symptoms are worse in the early hours about 4-5.00am, also from dairy products and cold air.

Kali carb   Exhaustion is a problem, the bad breath due to chronic indigestion associated with a high intake of sugars which ferment. Symptoms are worse in the early night hours.

Nux vomica   There are recurrent indigestion problems, mainly caused by too much rich fatty food or alcohol. The temperament is short-fuse and irritable.

Sulphur   The breath is foul, the tongue yellow or brown coated. There is indigestion with a gassy diarrhoea and flatulence. Recurrent skin infections of all types occur. There is an insatiable appetite.

BED WETTING

Because of bladder and psychological immaturity, some adolescents fail to gain full control over urine control at night and there may be a continuation of an infantile problem into the early teenage years. Although for many bed-wetters the problem does resolve in late childhood or the early teens, when it does continue longer, it is particularly distressing for the young pre-adult and needs to be handled in a particularly sensitive way by the parents.

At this age it is probably best to let the adolescent be responsible for washing his own sheets and bed-linen, making his own bed and if possible, having his own room. If he is treated as a mature person he will tend to relate to this and to become more mature. If he is chided and complained at, treated as a child by the parent - he will tend to stay one. Let the adolescent chart his own progress, encouraging him when there are dry nights and not being critical or making a comment when he is wet.

He should be encouraged to reduce the intake of fluids, especially in the late evening, trying to sleep less deeply and to train himself to wake when his bladder feels full, possibly using an ordinary alarm to wake him well before the time he usually wets. I recommend a light evening meal and to avoid alcohol, encouraging him to mix socially and to have a broad experience of others within his peer group, both male and female. The problem often completely resolves with his first sexual interest and involvement. The family should do everything they can to overcome any problem of shyness that may be present.

Remedies to consider:

Causticum   Indicated for the teenager who is a slow learner, with chronic catarrhal problems such as sinusitis. Rheumatic pains are also common.

Equisetum   A remedy for recurrent bladder problems. Sleep is too deep and the teenager does not wake from a full bladder. They often have nightmares which is a pointer to underlying emotional problems.

Lycopodium   For the immature teenager who presents himself as confident and mature. Relationships with his peer group and teachers are usually disturbed and learning is often impaired by high anxiety levels, especially any new unfamiliar situation. The intake of chocolate and sweet foods tends to be high and this should be reduced.

Pulsatilla   For the immature anxious teenager, who lacks confidence in himself. Bladder control is poor and he is easily tearful, without thirst, always worse for heat.

Sulphur   For recurrent bladder problems.

BEHAVIOUR PROBLEMS

These are common during the adolescent years with typical rebellion against authority figures, ideas, often difficult or aggressive, with independent behaviour. In some cases the rebellion does not occur and the teenager is over-compliant and shy or withdrawn, but this can be as much of a problem for the family as the healthier more overt challenging aggression.

Because adolescents come from a new and different social background from their parents and teachers, it is inevitable that they see things differently and in many ways what they see is correct and very positive. Their problem is often lack of skill as how best to present this within the framework of the family, school, or college. Because of their lack of experience and immaturity, coupled with a natural resistance of adults, to be told anything by a teenager, is often resented, seen as bumptious and inexperienced. As a result their contribution tends often to be undervalued and the teenager resents this. They have a natural tendency to either push their viewpoint on others, or to withdraw it and to act out their resentment and independence in other ways, often outside the family. Many of these are very healthy and positive, as often seen in sport or art.

Every adolescent needs to learn how to express his feelings and perceptions. When he presents them forcibly and over-vigorously it does not work, and he then feels rejected or misunderstood. This leads to a sense of alienation from the family, of not being loved or wanted. He tends to seek acceptance in his own peer groups and satisfaction in his new-found independence, from alcohol, smoking, drugs and sexual involvements.

Remedies to consider:

Lycopodium   Much of the problem is centred around being too eager, over hasty, off-balance emotionally in most of life's situations. The typical teenager is pseudo-mature, old before his years, anxious to please, but not thinking through sufficiently the consequences of his actions. He has spontaneity, but it is high-risk, and he is always in scrapes.

Nux vomica   The main behavioural difficulty is of poorly controlled, over-intense, too violent emotional responses to all situations. He is quick to flare up with a short-fuse disposition in almost any situation.

Pulsatilla   The shy disposition often hides a great deal of rage and dissatisfaction in life, hiding needs, vulnerability and libidinal drives under a blanket of shame.

Silicea   The problem is weakness both physically and psychologically. Thin and chilly, he is vulnerable to every infection, with recurrent throat or chest infections. But he is most hampered by a lack of confidence, avoiding competition or new social situations.

BLUSHING

One of the most troublesome of teenage problems, coupled with shyness, intense feelings of self-awareness, and often guilt. It is frequently linked to a repressive childhood and lack of experience with other adults and children of both sexes. Sometimes the parents have been too strict, or socially isolated, not free enough in their openness of communication and spontaneity with the child. Blushing has its roots in childhood immaturity and blockage of a healthy broad social development. In many cases the parents are shy with each other, or have been during their own childhood and adolescence. They may not be confident to handle the child's natural explorative behaviour, questions and spontaneity. All of this may cause uneasy guilt feeling and blushing in adolescence.

Most blushing is centred around repression or denial of the normal adolescent sexual drive and interests. The teenager is terrified of blushing, being the centre of attention or noticed, yet he also wants to be seen and often loves the limelight. The blush is a painful expression of shame, a signal that sexual thoughts and awareness are present, with needs for attention and to be noticed. The adolescent needs to be reassured that some shyness occurs in all teenagers. It is helpful for him to know that his parents also experienced shyness and were able to come to terms with it.

Sexual interest including masturbation is best treated in a natural way, as part of growing up. Shyness should not be ignored completely nor made a major issue. In this way, the adolescent is reassured, can relax more, feel less guilty and the problem will slowly resolve.

Remedies to consider:

Belladonna When shyness is linked to restless behaviour and overactivity. Anxiety is marked in all social situations, often with panic and severe anxiety.

Lycopodium The major problem is anticipatory anxiety, 'crossing bridges before they are met', expecting the worst catastrophe to occur. He needs enormous reassurance and constant proof of being valued and important. Confidence is weak, due to early emotional damage.

Pulsatilla A remedy for variable moods, and changeable self-confidence. He is often withdrawn with adults or unfamiliar social situations, but can also be dominating and aggressive to a weaker or younger child.

Silicea The teenager feels vulnerable, physically and psychologically.

Sulphur He is confused about his true feelings and motivations, with a tendency to be untidy in most of life's situations which then has repercussions on his psychological confidence.

BODY ODOUR

This may be a problem for adolescents who sweat profusely, or sometimes have an infection. The best treatment is scrupulous attention to personal hygiene and a constitutional treatment to improve overall health. Any localised focus of infection needs to be treated including those problems involving the sexual organs.

The diet should also be well-balanced, not too greasy or high in carbohydrates and with plenty of raw vegetables and fruit, also high in fibre. Regular exercise is also required for proper elimination by the adolescent. In some adolescents there is no pronounced body odour other than what is normal for the individual and healthy teenager. Female body odour is often related to the particular phase of her cycle. Where there is concern or preoccupation with normal body odour, it is often related to anxiety and fear of being rejected, or feelings of inadequacy.

Although the symptom is put forward at a physical level, where the root cause is emotional it is always linked to problems of basic trust and acceptance, often as much acceptance of self as well as others. If persistent and obsessional, it may indicate a more profound psychological state or mental illness that needs specialised care because of a possible delusional psychotic (break with reality) or depressive problem which it is reflecting. In many adolescents with this problem, there is an anxiety component present, and it is important that this is dealt with, preferably by the family or with help from the doctor, perhaps with some targeted or focused counselling, to prevent it developing into a more severe preoccupation.

Remedies to consider:

Carbo veg   There is gastric distention, the underlying cause of the problem related to a digestive problem.

Mercurius   The skin is covered with an offensive perspiration. Weakness and recurrent infection of the skin occurs, because of lowered vital resistance.

Natrum mur   The skin is greasy, or covered with sweat. Many of the problems are associated with an excessive intake of salt.

Nux vomica   The major cause is related to poor digestive functioning, often the result of an excessive intake of either alcohol or spicy foods. A sour nausea with flatulence is typical, also constipation.

Sulphur   For long-standing problems, usually associated with chronic digestive disorders. There is an excessive indiscriminate intake of food and offensive discharging skin infections.

BOILS

These are common in teenagers on any part of the body and often very painful. They are common on the face, neck, or back and on any area that is greasy and constantly being touched and rubbed or handled by the teenager and causing a secondary infection.

A major factor is an artificial diabetes caused by a diet which is too high in carbohydrates and providing a rich breeding ground for pus-making bacteria to flourish within the skin. If the adolescent is actually diabetic, then boils are already a potential problem and it is even more important to pay careful attention to the diet and keeping urinary and blood sugar at target levels. Boils are best treated keeping the diet low in all sugars, including chocolate, sugar alternatives such as saccharine, and also fruit because of the fructose (fruit sugar) content.

Scrupulous attention must be paid at all times to personal hygiene. A daily shower, morning and evening in hot weather, is preferable to taking an occasional bath and helps prevent infection. Recurrent boils are often associated with teenage acne (see section and advice on page 16). If severe, a boil may become persistent, eventually forming a deep painful discharging cavity or carbuncle. It is best to try to prevent this happening by paying careful attention to the diet and starting homoeopathic treatment early before the condition becomes chronic.

Remedies to consider:

Antimonium crud For recurrent severe problems with thickening, redness and irritation, worse from heat, especially in bed.

Hepar Sulph For cracked skin, which is unhealthy and tends to become infected and to discharge pus. The condition is aggravated by touch or cold air, but improved from warm applications.

Pulsatilla For recurrent boils or infected styes, often due to an excessive sugar intake and binge eating of cakes or chocolate. Symptoms are always very variable and emotional outbursts and tears are common.

Silicea For chronic problems with cracking of the skin, also recurrent infections. The nails crack or split easily and become infected. Cracks are common at the finger tips.

Sulphur For recurrent boils, usually associated with a high sugar intake and diarrhoea. All symptoms are worse for contact with water and for heat. The skin looks grey, greasy and dirty.

41

BULLYING

This is a common form of psychological abuse which damages the confidence of the bullied child and is liable to result in him failing to achieve his full potential. Many parents know that their child is being bullied but fail to prevent it happening. Any child may be bullied, but in particular, a child who is overweight, excessively small or tall may be picked upon, also where a child is nervous or of timid disposition. Bullying is less common where a child has a clearly defined physical or mental handicap. The bullied child is usually the victim in many situations, including the home, where he may take on a passive role. There are frequent problems in expressing aggression freely and he can usually only express anger through others. Because so much of his drive is suppressed, he tends to be unpopular, is picked upon or criticised.

Once the child develops more confidence and the parents show more interest and attention in his particular needs, patterns can change and his innate strengths and defences then emerge. Before this happens, he must first emerge as a person and an individual, able to disagree, to say 'no', to assert his own personality more and his particular perception of the world around him. When the family are able to tolerate more open communication and to allow a give- and- take situation, this leads to a re-structuring of the family dynamics and a previously subdued and timid teenager can emerge much more able to look after himself. Where he is taught judo or the martial arts to help build him physically, the individual attention he gains through the interest of the teacher and the parents, gives as much strength and confidence, as the classes.

Remedies to consider:

Lycopodium

To some extent he provokes bullying by his provocative manner and lack of confidence which makes him appear fearful. He is a loner, but likes to feel that others are in the vicinity. He is preoccupied with fantasies, rather than taking part in peer group play, preferring the company of older teenagers or adults which reinforces his pseudo-maturity, but does little for his actual confidence.

Pulsatilla

This teenager hides under a cloak of shame and inferiority, refusing to join in with the others and too easily provoked into tearful outbursts. He expresses rage, frustration and anger indirectly, through others, but when he does feel safe, and there are no adults around, he can also be very aggressive and bullying.

Silicea

For the small teenager, who is thin and underdeveloped, lacking confidence, drive and aggression. He tends to back-off when teased, provoked or confronted and because of his size and lack of confidence in himself, he is quickly picked upon and bullied.

43

CLAUSTROPHOBIA

Fear of restricted spaces is always a symptom of tension and anxiety . The fear of being confined reflects inner needs and feelings, including a tendency to avoid a possible hurt or rejection by hiding emotion, especially feelings of vulnerability.

Panic attacks tend to occur in situations which are threatening, for example, fear of open spaces, or agoraphobia. There is an underlying lack of confidence experienced as phobic anxiety. This should be dealt with as soon as symptoms occur, to prevent a rigid behaviour pattern becoming established. If the condition is left it may eventually limit social contacts, experience and emotional growth.

Typical fears are of travelling in lifts, the underground, centre seats in a cinema, theatre, or aeroplane, or any social situation where the teenager feels caught-up and trapped. Having to talk to people, to reply, be polite, meetings, job interviews, examinations, queues in a supermarket, all become places of threat and terror because he feels vulnerable or unable to cope or escape.

The basic conflict is often a strong need to control all feelings and needs, contrasting with powerful wishes to be more open, spontaneous and direct. Being able to be critical and standing up to authority (parental) figures are the most frequent areas of unresolved conflict.

Remedies to consider:

Argentum nit   Indicated where phobic problems are predominant. There is an aggravation of panic and fear when exposed to heat.

Aconitum   For acute problems with fear of impending collapse or death. Restlessness with anticipatory anxiety is also a feature.

Natrum mur   For long-standing problems with anxiety and lack of confidence. Depression with tearfulness is characteristic of this remedy.

Nux vomica   A useful remedy for spasms of anxiety, with irritability and either depression or sudden impulses to violence.

Phosphorus   The teenager is thin, pale and extremely nervous, lacking confidence. He is restless and over-sensitive in all forms of relationship.

COLDS, RECURRENT

The viral common cold is probably the most familiar illness and at some time affecting every adolescent. The virus is often seasonal and epidemic, but in the adolescent, two major factors are their lack of respect for a change in the weather and failure to be adequately protected by warm clothing (as part of adolescent fashion, invulnerability and omnipotence).

Typical symptoms involve the nose and throat, often the upper respiratory tract with catarrh, a sore throat and cough, associated with feelings of exhaustion and malaise. Because it is so frequent, no one can be totally immune from the common cold, but it is important that the adolescent takes reasonable precautions when the weather turns colder or damp to prevent a chill occurring and also if they have a cold, to be at least reasonably covered up to give some protection against a chest infection.

If recurrent, it may be associated with a lowered vitality and resistance, sometimes associated with a poor diet and also smoking, which reduces level of vitamin C. Antibiotics do not affect the condition and often only serve to kill off normal bowel flora, adding to the misery of the condition with diarrhoea and feelings of jaded exhaustion.

There is no evidence that taking extra vitamins or supplements of any kind, helps prevent the condition or shorten the period of discomfort. It is far better to keep resistance levels high by consistently eating foods which are naturally high in vitamins, taking care to eat some fresh fruit and raw vegetables daily.

Remedies to consider:

Aconitum For very acute colds with a raised temperature, often rigors with shivering. Anxiety is usually marked a marked feature.

Allium sat For colds with sneezing, the eyes red and irritated, with a profuse 'tap-like' clear watery discharge.

Arsenicum For acute colds when the teenager feels ice-cold, tired or exhausted and craving warmth. The chest is often involved, with an irritable cough, small amounts of frothy sputum.

Bryonia For acute colds with a dry irritating cough. The is throat dry, with a severe headache, worse for sudden jolting movements.

Influenzinum For acute viral colds.

Spongia tost Indicated for colds with a dry cough, fatigue and exhaustion.

CONCENTRATION, POOR

This is a common teenage problem and it is always important for the family to try to clarify the exact causes. If allowed to continue, it can lead to anxiety and failure to achieve full potential. The condition may be physical or psychological in origin. Physical conditions which undermine concentration include any infection or allergic condition, particularly if chronic or recurrent. Recurrent sinus problems with headache is often a cause, also severe hay-fever, eczema, asthma, allergic rhinitis or chronic nasal blockage of allergic origin. Failure to sleep from any cause including:- traffic noise, low background hum, vibration, or social irritations, causes fatigue and contributes to the problem.

Psychological factors which undermine concentration, include anxiety from any source, but particularly before an examination or interview, or any situation where the adolescent feels vulnerable and that he may not perform as well as he would wish. Any new or different change in the family dynamics tends to undermine the confidence and authority of the teenager. A change of partner by one of the parents is a frequent cause of friction with anxiety and concentration problems because of feelings of rejection, suspicion, mistrust, resentment, or dislike. It is important for parents to realise, that where changes occur within parental relationships - either a separation, or a new partner moving into the home, often with step-children, this creates a threat to the teenager. It is essential that ambivalent feelings are tolerated and accepted, allowed to be openly expressed and seen as a quite normal reaction for the adolescent.

Remedies to consider:

Lycopodium   For a 'butterfly mind', with constant distraction by outside events, or his own particular preoccupations at the time. Much of the problem is related to an underlying insecurity and fear of failure if he asserts himself, or is at all competitive. There is usually a long-standing insecurity problem which is the real root-cause of his problems and failure to reach his potential.

Pulsatilla   Concentration is often weak because this particular teenager is so changeable, varying from day to day, often hour to hour in his interests, involvement and emotional commitment. Because he is typically shy and nervous,he rarely gives full attention to any project. Often a gifted student, he is rarely consistent in the quality or output of his work.

Natrum mur   The teenager is anxious and a worrier, finding concentration difficult. Tension and nervousness are often the underlying factors in his focusing and learning difficulties.

CONSTIPATION

Infrequent bowel actions are often due to faulty bowel habits and training from childhood. Constipation is always a depressing and troublesome symptom for the adolescent. If the problem is dealt with by taking laxatives rather than finding out the causes, this tends to further entrench the problem.

Some of the major causes are dietary, with too much convenience food, high in refined flour and white sugar and lack of sufficient cereal and vegetable roughage in the diet. Lack of exercise is another cause especially if the teenager is house-bound.

Most cases are due to failure to establish a regular morning elimination reflex, or emptying the bowel as soon as there is an impulse to do so. Other causes are an inadequate intake of fluids, especially in hot weather, or where the adolescent is exercising and losing fluid by sweating but not replacing it.

Social factors are important, often occurring on holiday or wherever the teenager feels less confident, uncomfortable with the toilet facilities provided, especially the more sensitive adolescent who needs privacy and quiet.

Every adolescent should train his bowels to open daily by natural means, and usually after breakfast. Regular exercise helps, but a daily high-fibre diet is the best way to keep regular, using a breakfast cereal with plenty of fibre roughage preferably without added sugar.

Remedies to consider:

Alumina   For constipation associated with a high dietary intake of aluminium, either from aluminium saucepans in the kitchen or high intakes of tea. Other causes are aluminium salts in proprietary preparations, when taken for prolonged periods. There is severe constipation, and even a soft stool is passed with difficulty. It is often associated with a depressive mood, a sensation that time drags by or passes too slowly. A dry skin and itchy eyes are other problem areas.

Bryonia   The stools are hard and large, the constipation aggravated by heat or movement.

Nux vomica   Only small amounts of stool are passed, due to ineffective pushing down. The whole bowel area feels uncomfortable and often painful. Nausea may occur and extre mood irritability.

Opium   For absolute constipation, the bowels not working for days or weeks. The motion is usually painful, in the form of hard round balls. Vague drowsy remoteness is also characteristic.

51

DANDRUFF

Flaking of the scalp causes the typical dandruff symptoms which can be so distressing to the teenager. A dry form of eczema is present, associated with unhealthy hair, because it lacks the normal oils secreted by the seborrhoeic glands of the scalp and as a result lacks shine, vitality and bounce.

Regular gentle scalp massage can help the condition, using a light oil, e.g. almond or walnut oil.

Change to a more healthy raw food diet with emphasis on eating plenty of raw vegetables and fruit and always avoid fried, greasy foods. Cigarette smoke should be avoided because it reduces the blood supply to the skin and hair follicle, prematurely aging the skin and hair, aggravating the condition.

Remedies to consider:

Arsenicum
The scalp is burning or itchy, and feels cold and dry. Irritation is usually worse at night after midnight. The scalp is both painful and sensitive, but especially after exposure to a cold dry wind. The whole head is covered with dry scales from the dandruff.

Badiaga
For severe dandruff conditions, the scalp sore and dry. The condition tends to be worse in cold weather and to improve with heat, as in summer.

Kali sulph
General health is not good, the teenager often overweight, exhausted. Headaches are common. There are many hair problems, including recurrent infection and dandruff.

Lycopodium
For scalp problems associated with a dry skin. The condition may be aggravated by a high sugar intake, especially chocolate which is often craved. A right-sided headache with tearing pains is common. Indigestion problems with flatulence may occur.

DENTAL CARIES

This is nearly always caused by eating food which is too high in sugars and failure to regularly brush and floss the teeth. Sticky plaque accumulates, on or between the teeth, allowing the bacteria which cause caries to flourish.

Regular dental check-ups are essential every six months during the teenage years, and a good relationship with the dentist is essential for continuity of dental care. The dentist should be relaxed and able to communicate, in this way also encouraging the teenager to be at ease.

With modern fluoride dental treatments, dental caries may eventually become a thing of the past. It is still essential however to keep to a healthy diet, to brush the teeth twice daily, preferably after each meal, but not excessively (to avoid damage to the enamel layer of the teeth) and changing a toothbrush as soon as the bristles show signs of wear (at least every three month). As nutrition improves, and the sugar habit is kept under control, the health of the teeth will also improve.

Homoeopathy helps improve the overall health of the teenager, and with it, the health of the gums and teeth. Regular gum massage is recommended, using the finger or a firm toothbrush and a weak saline (salt) solution. It is also useful for toothache, gum infection (acute or chronic) and for painful root abscess problems.

Remedies to consider:

Apis
A remedy for toothache when there is swelling of the gum, the local area, red and tender. There is an absence of thirst. The symptoms are aggravated by hot drinks or touch.

Arnica
The area is red, swollen and feels bruised as if it has been kicked.

Belladonna
The local gum area is red and fiery, with throbbing pain, the teenager restless and anxious, worse for cold air or touching the area.

Chamomilla
For very severe dental conditions with irritability, the pain aggravated by hot drinks or any form of local heat. The cheek is often red and inflamed over the infected tooth.

Magnesium carb
There is severe toothache, with a tearing type of pain, worse at night and from cold air.

Plantago
For toothache which is improved by eating. The cheek is red and swollen. All symptoms are worse for cold draughts or touch.

DEPRESSION

This is a common problem for many adolescents as they can easily feel confused about themselves, out of touch with their inner directions and drives. Whenever a part of the self is suppressed it causes damage, because it feels as if lost or dead. Difficulties often centre around denied negative feelings towards a parent or sibling, felt to deny them the understanding, appreciation, affection and love they need. Often there is a long-standing conflict within the family, allowed to drift on without resolving it, or there is a basic failure to communicate.

In many instances the problems have evolved and changed, but the negatives still remain, from rigid viewpoints or judgments and often adopted many years ago. This can lead to a trapped, hopeless, blocked feeling. A young person may feel that things can never change, there is no way out, often that adults will never see him as he really is, give him a chance or a way out of an what feels to be an impasse. A combination of resentment and blockage within a stalemate situation, causes feelings of despair and depression. Suicidal thoughts or impulses may be present, but these are also close to feelings of need, loneliness, anger, resentment, or sometimes revenge.

Most teenagers need some help with their inner feelings when these are negative, especially when he feels hurt and misunderstood by those in authority.

Open communication and discussion of depression is essential, preferably within the family. When this is impossible, or cannot be tolerated, perhaps because feelings are too strong, or emerge as threatening or disturbing, then the problem is best dealt with by skilled counselling, combined with homoeopathic treatment.

Remedies to consider:

Arsenicum

For recurrent depressive problems, in a rigid, solitary, obsessional character. Most of the symptoms are worse in the early hours, particularly after midnight.

Aurum met

For severe suicidal depression with hopeless despair. Palpitations may be present due to anxiety.

Lycopodium

For depression and immaturity, in a teenager who has never fully been able to express himself, full of fears about what may happen in the future.

Natrum mur

A remedy for long-term depressive problems with rigidity of attitude, poor physical health and exhaustion. All symptoms are either better or worse from sea air. There is usually a high dietary salt intake.

Pulsatilla

For the shy immature passive teenager who tends to opt out of any social situation which poses a challenge, or is unfamiliar. Frequent weeping, with variation of mood is characteristic. There is intolerance of heat in any form.

DIARRHOEA

This may be of physical or emotional causation. The commonest physical causes are either dietary or infection. If too much food is taken at any one time, especially of a kind that does not suit the individual, then diarrhoea is a perfectly natural and healthy reaction to eliminate. Often food eaten by adolescents is not fresh, or has been frozen, thawed and refrozen, allowing bacterial entry. Infection may be caused by lack of hygiene, the food itself infected, or the standard of preparation before eating was not adequate.

All adolescents should pay scrupulous attention to personal hygiene whenever they consume food and be careful that the food they eat is well prepared and of good quality. Most cases of diarrhoea are of an infective nature and clear quickly within a few days. If symptoms persist, a doctor should be consulted to check the exact cause. Drink plenty whenever there are diarrhoea symptoms, and eat light, easily digestible food, until the condition passes. Food poisoning should be suspected if symptoms are severe and there is a temperature. Emotional reasons for diarrhoea are many and whenever there is anticipatory nervousness, fear, lack of confidence, a loose bowel movement may occur, especially before an interview or examination. If there is blood on the stool, colitis is a possibility and a doctor should be consulted.

After a bowel action, every adolescent should be encouraged to wash his hands thoroughly, including the nail areas with soap and a brush. This is even more important whenever he is preparing food.

Remedies to consider:

Natrum sulph

Indicated for loose watery diarrhoea, the stool yellow, worse in the morning and after damp weather.

Podophyllum

Helpful in chronic diarrhoea problems without pain, worse in the morning, from eating fruit and from heat.

Phosphoric acid

For painless diarrhoea with complete exhaustion. The stool is watery with much gassy flatus.

Pulsatilla

This remedy is of value where symptoms are intermittent and variable, the stool is loose, yellow or green, all symptoms worse for heat or fatty foods.

Sulphur

For severe recurrent morning diarrhoea which is offensive, with violent gassy flatus.

ECZEMA

Eczema is an acute or chronic skin reaction associated with redness, itchy irritability, swelling or oozing. The skin may crack, become thickened and is usually dry. The condition varies in extent, but tends to be localised around the face, back or inside of the ears, on the scalp, neck, chest or back, arms or legs, usually worse in the crease or flexure areas.

The causes are often unknown. A family hereditary factor may sometimes play a role, but other contributory causes, such as diet and emotion, are also important for eczema sufferers. When treated by steroids the eczema often stays just controllable, but in a chronic form, which can be seen or felt just under the skin. As soon as steroids are stopped, the eczema tends to erupt again with a more severe reaction.

In most teenage eczema problems, it is important to eliminate foods which the teenager is sensitive to, and which provoke an aggravation of the condition. These usuallly include chocolate, sweet cakes or confectionary, sugary drinks, milk, sometimes meat.

There is often an initial aggravation reaction at the start of homoeopathic treatment, as the remedies highlight the true nature of the eczema as they start working. In most cases the results are very good and a cure is achieved after a few months of treatment. It is always important to look at any underlying emotional factors which may cause low self-esteem and impaired confidence.

Remedies to consider:

Apis The area is red, painful, swollen and very tender to touch. The teenager is restless, without thirst, and worse from heat.

Bryonia The skin is hot and painful aggravated by movement or local heat.

Graphites Where there is oozing of a clear or straw-coloured fluid.

Petroleum The skin is dry, rough like sandpaper, tends to crack and is very irritating. Bleeding due to scratching is common and often leads to secondary infections.

Psorinum The skin is dry and intensely irritating The area has a dirty or grey appearance, all symptoms worse from cold air and better for warmth.

Rhus tox The eczema is red, thickened and very irritating, improved by warmth, fresh air and movement.

Sulphur For long-standing chronic problems, usually with infection, oozing and a thick offensive discharge.

EXAMINATION FEARS

Panic before an examination does not only reflect a sense of feeling unprepared for the particular task ahead, it is much deeper than that. In many students, fear occurs because of anticipatory anxiety, fearing not being able to respond or cope on the day, with feelings of doubt about confidence and adequacy to give of his best in a situation of pressure and appraisal.

The panic is often felt in other areas too, especially situations where he feels at a disadvantage, exposed, or 'on view'. It also occurs where he feels judged, or may be seen unfavourably rather than in a positive light.

Many teenagers are anxious, expecting failure and rejection. This is often part of his overall approach to new challenge situation, doubting his ability to cope and to be adequate, because he is over-critical of himself.

In some teenagers this is because there has been an over-critical parent or teacher, sometimes a grandparent who has undermined the confidence of the child. In others this is not apparent and no direct link is obvious, although the child may at an earlier date have had his confidence weakened, by a period of alienation or separation, from one or both parents. Sometimes there has been a loss through illness or death. The results from homoeopathy are usually very positive.

Remedies to consider:

Argentum nit   Where phobic anticipatory anxiety is extreme with terror of failure. The temperament is usually very controlled, obsessional and preoccupied with neatness and order. There is intolerance of heat which aggravates anxiety.

Gelsemium   For milder types of problems, with a tendency towards the dramatic and a basic insecurity. Apathy with exhaustion occurs, also anxiety aggravated by thunder.

Natrum mur   Indicated for more severe psychological anxiety states with deep insecurity and immaturity. Depressive problems are common. Attitudes towards change tend to be rigid.

Lycopodium   A remedy for the immature teenager who lacks social confidence. He has an enormous fear of failure and rejection, tending to shun all competitive situations and this is true for academic events as well as sport. His eventual career may not reflect his true ability, and he may opt for a safe backwater job where competition is minimal.

FIRST AID

Some first aid problems are unavoidable because all healthy adolescents like to extend themselves and test out every situation to the limit. Inevitably some spills and accidents occur. Homoeopathy is helpful and quick in action for most of these situations and especially valuable for cuts and grazes, bruised areas and sprains. Many of the common first-aid injuries of adolescents are sports-related, and need early treatment to prevent permanent damage causing limitation or pain in later years.

A rest period is essential after any injury, especially a sprain, painful twist, or joint injury, waiting until all pain and discomfort has ceased before resuming the strain of training and full activity. If in doubt, always obtain a medical opinion on any injury or area of persistent pain.

Prevention is always the best treatment. Begin all periods of training and activity with stretching exercises, and then a gentle warm-up, paced and rhythmic without straining, even when extending himself at full speed.

Use Arnica for all areas of painful swelling, with bruising, Ruta for tendon injuries, Hypericum for shooting pains, Calendula for cuts and grazes. A cold ice pack is helpful for swollen tendons or joints, or soaking the area in a cold saline (salt) solution. If pain or discomfort persists, try a wet pack treatment, wrapping a strip of damp cotton cheesecloth around the area, covering it with a dry towel until it dries out. Wash the cheesecloth after use each time, and repeat twice daily, until all discomfort has cleared.

Remedies to consider:

Arnica
A major remedy for ligament or soft tissue damage, especially where there is shock, bruising pain and swelling. The area affected is often black and blue from blood vessel damage and bleeding into the neighbouring tissues.

Bellis perennis
Another useful remedy for muscular damage with soreness and bruising. It is especially of value for a sprain, e.g. ankle or wrist after a fall. All symptoms are better for heat and firm binding.

Rhus tox
For damage and bruising of joints, ligaments and tendons, with pain and stiffness of the affected parts. All symptoms are relieved by heat and movement.

Ruta
Useful for tendon damage with stiffness, especially bruising of the flexor tendons of the wrist. It is useful where large joints are bruised, or the shins are painful after a kick or a fall. All symptoms are aggravated by cold or dampness.

GLANDULAR FEVER

An acute viral infection with painful enlargement of the lymphatic glands and spleen. There is severe fatigue and weakness, loss of drive and appetite, constipation and impaired concentration. The illness is common in adolescence, occurring at an any age, but particularly in the late teenage years.

There are often several cases of the illness occurring at the same time in a school, university, or college, the teenager particularly prone to glandular fever when tired, convalescent or under pressure. Diagnosis is often difficult, and the specific serum tests for antibodies not always positive.

The condition sometimes lasts for months, with a jaded loss of interest and a need to rest for long periods, closely resembling the chronic fatigue and exhaustion of the 'M.E.'syndrome. Glandular fever responds well and positively to homoeopathy. The full cure may however take several months and improvement is slow, because vitality is severely depleted by the infection.

Remedies to consider:

Baryta carb   Often indicated where there are large glands palpable in the neck area. Recurrent acute throat infections may be a feature of the illness. Improved by walking and fresh air.

China   Where exhaustion and near collapse is the main problem. Intermittent peaks of raised temperature occur. All symptoms are aggravated by exposure to draughts and being touched.

Nux moschata   Where exhaustion and fatigue are the major symptoms, usually feeling chilled and with a tendency to fainting or drowsiness.

Phosphoric acid   A further remedy to consider for the typical exhaustion of this condition, with listless apathy and extreme fatigue from any form of exercise or concentration. They feel better for warmth and are intolerant of cold air or damp.

The specific glandular fever nosode or homoeopathic vaccine equivalent.

GROWING PAINS

These are common in teenagers and sometimes occur in younger children. They are of unknown origin, but thought to relate to changes in the long bones as growth spurts occur.

The main symptoms are aching discomfort in the limbs, often at rest, but sometimes following physical activity, especially if it has been strenuous. The child should be reassured and if persistent should be checked by a doctor to exclude any other causes of the symptoms. Smoking should be avoided, as it may aggravate the problem.

It is always important to ensure that every teenager has an adequate supply of protein for muscle growth and repair at this time, also adequate calcium in the diet. There should be some daily exposure to fresh air, light, and sunshine.

Teenagers should not be encouraged to stay indoors all the time watching television or a computer video screen. If the condition is aggravated by field sports, such as football or cross country events, these should be stopped until the symptoms subside. During this time, an alternative sport is often possible, such as swimming.

Remedies to consider:

Calcium phos   For long bone pains in the tall and
                     thin teenager who is always
                     chilly. Symptoms are worse when
                     there is a change of barometric
                     pressure, usually improved by
                     warmth. The teenager craves
                     highly seasoned or savory acid
                     foods, such as pickles, which may
                     aggravate the problem.

Gelsemium   Cramps, weakness, or intermittent
                     pains are common, the legs weak
                     and tired after only mild exercise.
                     All symptoms are aggravated by
                     damp and cold conditions.

Hypericum   Indicated where there are darting
                     pains, which move up the limbs,
                     sometimes accompanied by cramp
                     in the calf muscles, or an irritating
                     tingling type of sensation. All
                     symptoms are worse for exposure
                     to cold or damp.

Rhus tox   For tearing aching limb pains,
                     sometimes associated with joint
                     swelling. Symptoms are improved
                     by heat and movement, but
                     aggravated by cold, damp and
                     immobility.

GROWTH, STUNTED

It is always a matter for concern, when a child fails to grow and reach his expected targets for height and weight. In some adolescents, the cause is a mineral deficiency, in others, inadequate nutrition, with lack of essential vitamins, unfortunately now common in many famine areas of the world.

It occurs less frequently in the UK, but may still happen in some immigrant communities where diet is severely restricted, or there is lack of exposure to sunlight. In others the cause is a genetic abnormality, with failure to take-up or absorb essential ingredients from the food. There may also be a metabolic or hormonal imbalance syndrome, usually of genetic origin.

In most cases, the condition is a continuation of a problem from childhood. Where it is of more recent origin, and the normal teenage growth spurt is not occurring, it needs careful investigation to clarify the cause. Any acute infection of the lungs, heart, or kidney, may stop the normal growth process, needing careful treatment and follow-up, to ensure, that after the illness, growth is stimulated to occur.

Homoeopathy encourages growth after an illness and poses no toxic risks for the patient. If a teenager is small but healthy, taking regular exercise and a diet that is perfectly adequate, he may be small for genetic reasons, particularly if one or both parents are also small. But any child who fails to be within his height and growth norms should be checked by his doctor as soon as the parents feel that there may be a problem.

Remedies to consider:

Baryta carb

Where the teenager has failed to mature and is delayed in all his developmental milestones. He is especially vulnerable to all infections, and has poor resistance, with endless colds, sinus infections and chronic throat or nasal catarrh. He is usually improved by walking and fresh air.

Silicea

For the teenager who fails to grow and fully mature physically. He is often vulnerable to recurrent throat and tonsillar infections and also tends to lack confidence and persistence in work and concentration. The feet often sweat. He is better for warmth and also humid conditions.

Tuberculinum

For long-standing growth problems, the teenager thin, pale, but at the same time energetic, liking change and travel. Exhaustion is often a problem, worse before a storm or change of barometric pressure, also from cold damp air, better for movement and fresh air.

GRUMBLING APPENDIX

The commonest symptoms are recurrent lower abdominal pains, griping and colicky. These are usually right-sided, but not associated with a raised temperature, or causing severe abdominal tenderness, nausea or vomiting. The adolescent is clearly in discomfort, but not severely ill and the pulse rate remains normal (72 per minute).

Often the bowels are constipated, and there is an absence of the normal adolescent interest in food.

If there is any doubt, it is important to have a medical opinion, to ensure that surgery is not overlooked or indicated.

In addition to the homoeopathic remedy, warm drinks are helpful and often a hot water bottle.

Remedies to consider:

Aconitum Abdominal pain is acute and colicky, the whole area tender to touch. Thirst is marked and loose stools are a feature. Pain is relieved by warm applications, but aggravated by lying on the right side.

Belladonna Sweating with restlessness is present, also nausea or vomiting. The whole abdominal area is sensitive and all symptoms are aggravated by coughing, jarring, or the least pressure from bedclothes.

Bryonia There are stitch-like lower abdominal pains, aggravated by movement, but relieved by warmth.

Mercurius Stabbing discomfort is present in the lower abdomen with sweating and diarrhoea. The abdomen is tender, worse for lying on the right side, also for heat.

Nux vomica Indicated where there are spasms of colicky pains with constipation. Irritability is marked.

HAIR-LIFELESS

Whenever hair lacks lustre and vitality it often means that the general health is impaired, or there is an internal imbalance, either physically, or psychologically. Often the hair is dry, the ends breaking. If the hair is lifeless, it is important to look at the diet, and to consider if there is a hormonal imbalance. The condition is improves when fats and carbohydrates, especially sugars are reduced. Other factors are a polluted home or office environment, particularly from dust or cigarette smoke.

The too frequent use of strong shampoos is damaging, and although the intention is to keep the hair clean and healthy, the result is often the reverse, and it loses all vitality, bounce and lustre. Unless they are working in a very dusty environment, most teenagers should not shampoo their hair more than once a week. Always use a pure herb-based natural shampoo, with a single wash and rinse the hair several times, preferably with rain water and then gently towel-dry. Most commercial shampoos contain strong chemical substances, and have a negative effect on the natural oils of the hair.

Avoid damaging the delicate hair follicles, by over-vigorous massage, or the prolonged use of a very hot hair dryer. Perms or colorants which contain strong chemicals should be avoided. Their use is not recommended if the hair is at all weak, lifeless, or the ends are splitting. If the ends are splitting, this should be removed, cutting the last half-inch of hair length. Gently massage the scalp weekly with almond oil.

Remedies to consider:-

Bryonia

For dry hair and scalp, with dislike of heat or movement. Mood irritability is usually present.

Kali sulph

The hair is thin and dry, the scalp unhealthy with dandruff.

Lycopodium

Indicated when the hair is thin, falls out easily, or there is premature baldness. Stress causes a craving for sugar leading to a high dietary sugar intake. This is often a major contributory factor to the problem.

Pulsatilla

The hair is thin and lifeless. A high dietary carbohydrate intake often aggravates the problem.

Silicea

For lifeless hair which lacks vigour and bounce. The nails also tend to split easily and there is a poor circulation. Sweating on the head may be a feature, also intolerance of cold air.

HAY FEVER

The common late spring or summer eye, nose, chest and sinus condition, usually due to a pollen allergy. Hay fever starts in May or June and may carry through until September, or later, depending upon the humidity, also trees, plants, and crops in the region.

The most common symptoms are a severe rhinitis with sneezing, a profuse watery discharge, conjunctivitis (red eyes), a sore throat, sometimes tightness of the chest. It is always an unpleasant condition for the sufferer, undermining confidence, concentration, and causing a low of energy.

The specific causes are often unknown, but it is usually due to pollen sensitivity and often quite specific.

Plants which may be involved are Rape seed, tree pollens (for example Silver birch), roses, various grasses. Allergy to a specific flower or pollen, once known, can be made up into homoeopathic potency, usually 3X or 6c.

In some teenagers, the condition starts much later, at the end of the summer in September, and is then due to sensitivity to moulds in the air, usually from trees. A few cases of teenage hay-fever are unrelated to the pollen count, occurring throughout the year and often severe on days when it is raining, or the count is minimal. The problem is usually increased by stress or emotional tensions, aggravating any tightness of the chest that is present. Contact with pets, and exposure to high levels of house dust, may also aggravate the problem.

Remedies to consider:

Arsenicum   For the teenager who is isolated or a loner with underlying relationship difficulties. Obsessional neatness may be present, and all symptoms are worse in the early hours after midnight. He is often very chilly and asthma may be an additional problem.

Ipecacuanha   Useful when there is associated nausea or vomiting.

Kali carb   Recommended when anxiety is marked with apathy or exhaustion. All symptoms are worse in the early night hours, especially at 4-5.00 a.m.

Nux vomica   Indicated for acute hay fever problems, worse at night and for stuffy atmospheres. Irritability with indigestion is often a marked feature.

Sabadilla   For hay fever with marked sneezing and a profuse clear nasal discharge. The eyes also water and are often red and swollen. All symptoms are aggravated by cold damp conditions.

HICCUP

Hiccup is due to repeated spasm of the diaphragm muscle and often associated with indigestion or alcohol. The cause is usually unknown. When recurrent it may be associated with a digestive problem or underlying emotional tension.

In most cases the symptom is unimportant, and does not reflect a severe underlying illness. It is only medically important if severe, prolonged or recurrent.

It tends to be helped by drinking sips of water or milk. The response to homoeopathy is usually very positive.

Remedies to consider:

Cuprum   Helpful for pre-menstrual hiccup which is improved by cold drinks. Nausea and colicky diarrhoea may also be present. The stomach gurgles loudly when liquids are taken.

Ginseng   Useful when the hiccup is associated with usually right-sided abdominal pain or discomfort, Gurgling of the lower abdomen is typically present.

Hyoscyamus   For the talkative rather suspicious teenager, with abdominal cramping or colicky discomfort. Flatulence may accompany hiccup, often food related or it may occur at night.

Nux vomica   Spasms of colicky abdominal pain occur with irritability, often worse after eating, or on waking. All symptoms are better for warm humid weather.

Sulphuric ac   Indicated for hiccup with exhaustion and sour indigestion. Nausea may be present, with a chilled stomach sensation. Most of the discomfort is improved by warmth.

IMMATURITY

To some extent, all adolescents are immature, because they are in a pre-adult phase of development. Although mature physically in their early teens, many are uncomfortable psychologically, feeling like a child locked into an adult body. Adolescents experience their relationships in an intense extreme way, reflecting ideals but not realities. They are still dominated by infantile parts of their emotional make-up, in much the same way as a young child and make demands for instant love, understanding, results, reactions and problem-solving. Waiting and delay is difficult for every teenager.

Because teenagers need constant reassurance, if a response is not forthcoming, or questioning, they tend to either reject it totally, or see themselves as a failure. Suddenly they are no longer buoyant and confident and become dejected or depressed. Mood swings and mood extremes, are common, also lack of confidence. Demands are even more volatile just before the female cycle begins, and often worse until it becomes regular and established. The best approach for parents is to stay calm, available, clarifying the realities of underlying anxiety, encouraging the teenager to talk rather than throw a tantrum or become irritable. Once the problem and any fears are brought down to size, seen in perspective, anxiety is relieved and just as quickly their mood changes again.

Parents should stay in touch with the kind of problems and emotions they themselves experienced as a teenager, able to share how they felt then and how they survived.

Remedies to consider:

Argentum nit   For phobic anxiety problems, causing withdrawal and social isolation.

Lycopodium   The teenager is tense and tends to rush and anticipate problems. This means that all experiences are emotional, not sufficiently experienced in depth or allowed to become a part of him.

Pulsatilla   For the adolescent who fears all closeness and involvement, so that life is kept superficial, at a safe distance in case of failure or rejection.

Silicea   For the thin, small, often pale underdeveloped adolescent who is fearful of failure or 'making a fool' of himself. Lack of confidence is the major problem, coupled with avoidance of others, especially competitive situations, leading to immaturity.

INDIGESTION

This is a common problem because adolescents tend to eat the wrong foods, and what they do eat, they eat too quickly. Because they are always in a rush, digestion time is minimal, and with the present popularity for fast food, their diet is too high in fats and sugars.

The commonest symptom is gassy flatulence, due to fermentation, causing a noisy intestine as it struggles to digest. Wind occurs, causing a sense of fullness or flatulence, and may erupt upwards or downwards, but it is usually unpleasant for the adolescent, and a source of embarrassment.

Adolescents don't like to feel dependent on anything or anyone and this includes food and the time it takes for digestion to take place. Indigestion is bound to occur, until the adolescent learns that food must be chewed well and eaten slowly.

Parents can help by setting a good example - eating slowly, allowing plenty of time for the family meal, and not encouraging television or radio at this time.

Remedies to consider:

Argentum nit   There is belching with flatulence and intolerance of heat. Panicky anxiety is often a feature.

Carbo veg   Useful for gassy upper abdominal flatulence with distention. Nausea with exhaustion is often a feature. All symptoms are better for movement and aggravated by lying down or inactivity, also from eating rich foods or wine, better from cool fresh air.

Lycopodium   For right-sided upper abdominal discomfort with heart-burn. Most of the symptoms are aggravated in the afternoon, or if a meal is missed or delayed.

Nux vomica   Helpful for colicky upper abdominal pains with nausea and irritability.

Sulphur   A remedy for gassy, offensive flatulence, with persistent hunger, even just after eating. Diarrhoea, colic, abdominal distention and lack of energy, are often present.

LYMPHATIC GLANDS, TENDER

This is essentially a healthy response to an infection anywhere in the body and reflects the defensive lymphatic system working to localise inflammation and prevent it from spreading.

If there is a throat infection, the lymph nodes of the neck are usually tender and often enlarged, feeling like hard nodules. The same is true if a toe or finger is infected, with tender lymph nodes in the groin or arm-pit.

Glandular fever causes a generalised enlargement of the lymphatic system, with tender nodes in several areas, including the spleen which is tender and frequently enlarged. Mumps also leads to painful very lymphatic swelling.

Where lymph nodes are persistently enlarged and not related to an obvious infection, a medical opinion should be sought in order to clarify the underlying cause. Often lymph nodes are palpable in the groin or elsewhere when a teenager is tired, low on vitality and with few energy reserves.

Every local skin infection should be treated properly, the area kept clean, and covered with a sterile dressing.

Remedies to consider:

Antimonium crud The tender glands are associated with an acutely inflamed throat which feels raw. There is a slimy yellow mucus discharge from the area affected. Laryngitis with loss of voice may also be a complication. All of the symptoms are improved by fresh air and rest, aggravated from eating acidic foods.

Baryta carb The throat and tonsils are infected with a thick yellow discharge and raised temperature. Swallowing is usually painful.

Hepar sulph Sharp splinter-like pains of the throat make swallowing difficult. All symptoms are aggravated by cold air and better from humid conditions and steam inhalations.

MASTURBATION

Masturbation is perfectly normal for all teenagers, as an expression of sexual drive, a source of pleasure and often relief from frustration and tension. Masturbation itself is not usually a problem, but sometimes misplaced guilt becomes associated with it and a cause of anxiety.

This is most common within a repressive, or rigid family, where all sexuality topics are taboo. Fortunately healthier attitudes are now more common and teenagers are able to read and talk about sexual matters more openly than a decade ago. This has led to a healthier approach to sexuality overall and guilt problems are fewer than a few years ago.

In some adolescents the problem is an inability to masturbate because of anxiety and guilt, which can be damaging if it becomes an obsessional preoccupation. There is still a need for parents to talk more openly with teenagers about sexual topics and many girls are still not informed about their cycle, why it is occurring and what it means, because their own mother is too shy and inhibited. In the same way fathers do not explain to their sons the normality of a 'wet dream' and how it relates to normal development.

All teenagers are curious and interested about their body in all its aspects, but especially their sexual development. At some time they have an interest in masturbation. This is healthy and normal. It is especially important that parents accept and understand this and do not condemn it or imply any links with guilt or abnormality.

Remedies to consider :

Argentum nit   Indicated for compulsive masturbation, associated with phobic-anxiety problems, also intolerance of heat.

Natrum mur   For deep-seated insecurity problems, where masturbation is an attempt to find comfort and reassurance. The teenager is usually ill at ease in all social situations and never able to feel natural or to relax fully.

Lycopodium   Of value where there are problems of anticipatory anxiety in an immature adolescent who has few friends. He is typically insecure and also accident-prone.

Pulsatilla   Recommended for the fearful, often painfully shy teenager with deep-seated confidence problems and sexual anxieties. He is often depressed and easily tearful needing constant reassurance as to his worth and value.

MIGRAINE

This is a distressing complaint, often of unknown origin. It is not uncommon for one of the parents to have recurrent headaches or some form of allergy, but migraine is not an inherited condition. The commonest symptoms are severe one-sided headaches, associated with nausea and sometimes stomach discomfort. They can come on at any time, but are often worse at period times, or whenever there is any situation of pressure or stress. There is frequently an underlying emotional factor present, with undeclared tension, anxiety, or lack of confidence. Food allergy, such as sensitivity to chocolate, oranges, tomatoes or wine, is also a common trigger to attacks.

One young teenager with a severe migraine problem, had reading difficulties at school. She was humiliated by her teacher, and treated as either lazy or a dunce. When dyslexia was finally diagnosed, she was moved to a special school for children with learning difficulties, and given intensive help with her reading problems. After eighteen months, her reading level reached the expected norm for her age and she became free of all migraine symptoms. She was then referred back to her original school, and again started to develop daily migraine, with stomach pains and nausea. When she was moved to a new class and a more sympathetic teacher, the migraines disappeared. In this child, the underlying emotional factors which were a trigger to her migraines, were anxiety, loss of confidence and fear of being confronted or humiliated.

The homoeopathic approach is usually helpful for the majority of migraine problems.

Remedies to consider:

Belladonna   For acute migraine, the face red and hot, worse for noise, bright lights, heat and jolting movement.

Carbo veg   A remedy for heavy or tight-band headaches, worse from rich foods or hot humid conditions.

Chionanthus Indicated for sick headaches of the forehead, often linked to the female cycle.

Gelsemium   Useful for dull heavy headaches, aggravated by touch or emotion.

Iris versic   For mainly right-sided forehead headaches associated with nausea, Most symptoms are worse in the evening.

Lachesis   There is a left-sided headache, with dizziness, worse on waking and aggravated by movement.

Natrum sulph The headaches are at the back of the head and accompanied by sweating of the scalp.

Psorinum   A useful remedy for headaches at night, the head feels as if it has been kicked. Dizziness is often present and hunger is persistent. Pain is worse in cold air.

MOOD CHANGES

These are quite normal for most teenagers, before emotional maturity is fully established. Changes in moods occur and for the least reason, not usually related to a particular reason. At that time a mood can suddenly alter from a high, feeling confident, attractive and buoyant, to a low of being a failure, unloved and unattractive. Tears are common, particularly before the female cycle, but equally a critical outburst may occur, with a flash of aggressiveness. Much of the reason behind such wild swings in mood is that the teenager is functioning at many different levels, and each level has its particular energy and intensity of emotion.

At any one moment the teenager may be involved, communicating and relating well, seemingly sensitive to deep issues, yet at the same time he may also be thinking of something different which seems trivial. Whatever the issues, he is never very far removed from his appearance, especially his hair, the clothes he is going to wear, or feeling hungry, usually for something sweet.

As he swings from one issue and need to another, so too do his moods and emotions. He may pass rapidly from being serious, to becoming flippant, provocative and childlike. The teenager is usually very aware of this, and often cannot explain or control it. He feels swept along by the storm of his needs and emotions as they occur, and often completely taken over by them. Only in retrospect can he look back and apologise, or wonder what came over him. Because of these swings, he is also easily influenced, and a prime target for the media, promoting cosmetics, alcohol and cigarettes.

Remedies to consider:

Argentum nit   Where mood changes are associated with obsessional fears and rigid attitudes. There is anxiety in all new situations and intolerance of hot stuffy environments.

Natrum mur   Recommended for the depressed moody teenager who is a loner and never at ease or natural in any social situation.

Nux vomica   A remedy for the over-intense and immature adolescent who is frequently depressed with sullen mood changes, especially with spasms of irritable frustration. Much of the underlying tension is also expressed through the intestinal canal, with chronic digestive and constipation problems, which adds to the irritability.

Pulsatilla   This remedy is for mood changes varying between laughter, dramatic attention - seeking behaviour, to tears of despair. There is immaturity of emotion causing uncertainty and anxiety in all social situations, with fear of the opposite sex and emotional closeness. Intolerance of heat.

NAIL BITING

Nail biting is common in many sensitive or anxious teenagers, reflecting tension and anxiety about more spontaneous self-expression. In most cases there is a fund of unexpressed aggression and resentment, that has never been talked about or discussed in any depth.

The typical adolescent is usually shy and fearful, and lacks confidence. Nail biting is an obvious expression of tension, but it often reflects a wish to make a more direct or biting comment. It is often an expression of suppressed anger, sometimes an attempt to disarm himself, because at a primitive symbolic level, the nails represent man's aggressive claws.

Because nail biting attempts psychologically to deny the individual his aggressiveness, encouraging passivity, it is harmful. It should be positively discouraged, the parents making every attempt to get the teenager to be more open and spontaneous about his feelings, including his anger. If the habit occurs when watching an exciting or violent action film or television scene, it is helpful if afterwards, the parents encourage discussion of his and their own reactions and feelings.

Attempts at spontaneity are likely to be slow at first, because of the strength of his fears and anxiety, usually of rejection or punishment. Spontaneity is vital for the healthy development and psychological growth of every adolescent.

Remedies to consider:

Lycopodium There is tension and anxiety which is not talked about, particularly fears of the future or a preoccupation with failure. The teenager appears mature and older than his years, but pays a heavy price for his pseudo-maturity by becoming isolated from his own peer group.

Pulsatilla The nail-biting is an expression of anger and a withholding. Much of the tension relates to shyness and frustration, particularly lack of confidence with the opposite sex. Self-destructive patterns of behaviour fuel the anger and blockage of spontaneity.

Natrum mur This type of teenager goes through life biting back upon himself, so that any form of social expression is always a partial one and inevitably frustrating.

Silicea The claws of spontaneity and confident self-expression are bitten back in case there is lack of control or he hurts or wounds another. There is an overall lack of confidence and depression.

NOSE BLEEDS

Nose bleeds or epistaxis, are often due to a blow, or there is irritation of the nasal passages, causing congestion and bleeding.

Nose picking of an itchy or dry area in the nasal orifice is a very common cause of the symptom. It may also be associated with an infection or develop spontaneously because of hot or humid conditions.

More rarely the causes are due to teenage blood-pressure, or there is a disturbance of the blood clotting mechanism because of sensitivity to a drug or medication, for example Aspirin. If the problem is recurrent, there may occasionally be a deeper disturbance, as occurs in haemophilia.

In most cases the problem responds well to homoeopathy and is only a temporary inconvenience. If it is a recurrent problem, the cause should always be clarified.

Remedies to consider:

Arnica When bleeding follows upon a blow, the area sore and bruised.

Belladonna For a spontaneous nose-bleed associated with congestion or fullness of the head or nasal area.

Bryonia For recurrent early morning nose-bleeds, often associated with a migraine headache. All symptoms are aggravated by heat or jolting.

China For nasal bleeding on getting up in the morning. Sneezing and recurrent febrile episodes.

Ferrum phos There is a flow of bright red blood from the nose, worse at night or early morning, on the right side and from touch or jolting.

Hamamelis There is a slow discharge of dark blood from the nasal area which does not clot easily.

Nitric acid A remedy for nose-bleeds associated with sharp stitch-like or splinter pains in the nasal area and typically worse at night.

Phosphorus For profuse bright red epistaxis in a sensitive but nervous teenager.

OBSESSIONS

Obsessional patterns in an adolescent, always reflect a preoccupation with order, excessive self-control and insecurity, as he attempts to control all the possible risks of life, fundamentally those of change and exploration, within the confines of the obsessions and rituals. For many teenagers, there has been a blow to confidence in early childhood, a loss, separation, or divorce, which made him vulnerable.

The obsessional problem is best discussed within the family, by the parents as soon as it becomes obvious. Try to clarify the situations where his obsessions are most active, how they link to any new situations, and how long they have taken to develop. The fears are usually illogical, perhaps a coming visit from someone who is much loved, can become a threat if he fears he may inadvertently cause damage or harm. Any safe and positive situation, may become a danger that threatens to take the parents or security away, the obsessional pattern, like a magical spell, that can bind and outwit an evil fate felt to be lurking just around the corner.

If severe, the obsessional problem, may limit social contacts, exploration and exposure, which are all essential for confidence and healthy development.
When the problem is long-standing, or severely restrictive, leading to isolation and distortion of others, it should be treated under medical supervision, using homoeopathic remedies to try to break down the rigid patterns. The family should encourage spontaneity and be relaxed and open themselves. Some individual counselling or psychotherapy may be required.

Remedies to consider:

Arsenicum   For phobic obsessional problems in a chilly teenager with circulation problems who shuns the company of others and is very rigid in all his attitudes and relationships. Exhaustion is often a typical feature.

Ignatia   Indicated for ritualistic anxiety problems linked to unresolved grief and loss, either recent or in the past. Depression is usually also present and a hopeless defeatist attitude to life.

Natrum mur   A useful remedy for rigid defensive attitudes to change. He is depressed, lacking energy because most of the vitality is taken up by obsessional preoccupations. Mood swings are common. There is a tendency to avoid others, felt to be a threat or to make a demand, which he feels unable to meet.

Phosphorus   A remedy for the tall, thin, pale and anxious teenager who has many obsessional-anxiety patterns. There is a constant need for reassurance and a conviction of impending loss or failure.

OVERSENSITIVITY

This may be a part of the individual temperament of the teenager. It is only important if extreme, leading to unhappiness or severe frustration. Some sensitivity is necessary and a positive valuable aspect of the personality, but when it becomes excessive or distorted, it becomes harmful.

The oversensitive teenager sees potential or implied criticism at every step or encounter, and this may lead to shyness or withdrawal. If severe it may lead to social isolation. Some rebuff in life is inevitable and every adolescent can be very sharp and direct with his comments and often hurtful. It is usually the already damaged adolescent who is most at risk of becoming oversensitive and seeing every comment as critical.

Oversensitivity is one aspect of shyness, which can be very painful, and damaging for the development of confidence. Parents can help by showing the teenager that his particular interpretation of an event may be either a partial understanding of what happened or sometimes totally incorrect. Also that not everyone is out to hurt or devalue him.

Whenever his anticipation of a relationship or social outing are proved wrong, this can be used positively to show how he distorts in a negative way, feeding the more oversensitive aspects of his personality. It is important to do this with sensitivity and understanding and not to criticise or apportion blame in any way.

Remedies to consider:

Argentum nit   There is fear of failure and the future with intolerance of heat.

Lycopodium   This teenager lacks confidence because everything he does in life lacks depth because it is done in a hurry. This leads to lack of confidence, often to criticism which adds feeling of inadequacy. Oversensitivity is increased by a tendency to be off-balance most of the time which creates accident-proneness.

Pulsatilla   For the shy, blushing, immature teenager who runs away from life and others because of guilt and shame. All feelings and moods are strong yet changeable, and even the oversensitivity varies.

Silicea   Useful for the teenager who is weak on determination and staying power in any situation where the outcome is uncertain, or where there is an element of competition. He is often thin and underweight and needs building-up physically as well as psychologically.

OVULATION, PAINFUL

Because of oestrogen hormone build-up at the time of ovulation, many adolescents experience mild, temporary, lower abdominal discomfort, or intermittent cramping pains. This is caused by a combination by muscular contraction of the fallopian tube, but also due to ligament spasm. At this time, the tube is pulled into the optimum position to receive the released ovum for fertilisation and a possible pregnancy to occur.

Another factor, may be slight ovarian bleeding as the egg is released, irritating the abdominal peritoneal cavity and causing temporary discomfort. The pain usually lasts for about one day. It is important to understand, that any discomfort felt, is not an illness and it should not be seen as a signal for alarm.

Homoeopathic treatment is usually effective, avoiding any possible side-effects. The conventional approach often recommends either analgesics (pain relievers) of the aspirin/codeine type, or sometimes the contraceptive pill is prescribed to inhibit ovulation.

Remedies to consider:

Colocynth   There are severe cutting or cramping pains at this time, worse for cold air and improved by local heat, as from a hot water bottle. Irritability and intolerance are usually marked features.

Lycopodium   For right-sided ovarian cramping pains.

Naja   The pain is mainly left-sided, worse from cold air, but improved by movement and exercise.

Nux vomica   Indicated for colicky, irregular, ovarian pains, with nausea and constipation. Irritability is marked.

Sabina   Recommended for severe ovarian pains, often felt down the front of the thighs and aggravated by heat or movement.

PERIOD PROBLEMS

PAIN

Painful periods are common during the adolescent years until ovulation and the menstrual cycle become fully established. It is perfectly usual for most teenage girls to experience some pain and cramp during the early cycles, and often intermittently for about a year.

The exact cause of the painful periods in adolescence is not always understood, but it is thought to be due to oestrogen insufficiency leading to imbalance and irregular hormone action. The imbalance causes cramping pains of the uterine muscles and an intermittent blood flow in the pelvic area, which leads to heaviness, dragging-down discomfort and sometimes clot formation.

Other theories relate the cause of the painful periods to another group of hormones, called prostaglandins, which in excess, cause uterine spasm and cramping pains. In some teenagers there may also be an underlying emotional or a family stress factor, which further contributes to period discomfort and pain.

Remedies to consider:

Belladonna   For dragging-down pain with heavy periods, often too early.

Chamomilla   Colicky pains, the periods dark with clots and heavy, with restlessness and irritability.

Coffea   The periods are early, often prolonged with clots. Restless irritability is a feature. Pains are relieved by local heat and lying down.

Magnesium phos   A useful remedy for colicky period pain, the periods often early with a dark loss. The pains are relieved by heat.

Nux vomica

For colicky pain, with extreme irritability, the periods irregular, early and prolonged.

Pulsatilla   For variable period discomfort, aggravated by any emotion or from heat, often associated with moody withdrawal or tears.

Sulphur   There is a thick dark menstrual loss with mild discomfort and sweating. All symptoms are aggravated by heat, contact with water and worse in the morning.

PERIOD PROBLEMS

IRREGULARITY

The exact cause is usually not known, but most modern theories relate the problem to hormonal imbalance and an inadequate oestrogen output. It is a common problem in adolescence, particularly during the first two or three years of the menstrual cycle.

The usual pattern, is a cycle which is unpredictable, the girl either completely missing a period, or it comes late. In some adolescents, the period may occur every two or three weeks, sometimes persisting like this for a few years, until the girl matures, gradually settling down into a 28 day cycle.

Pain is often absent, the loss either light or scanty, sometimes heavy with clots, but usually fairly consistent in the amount of loss. Some adolescents may only experience a minimal loss on some cycles, with slight spotting for a day or two and then nothing until the next cycle begins. Quite often a period is delayed for about two weeks, before it occurs, to be followed by a normal 28 day cycle, and then another two week gap followed by a loss.

If the periods are both frequent and heavy, the adolescent may become tired and exhausted, sometimes anaemic. If this occurs, an iron-replacement treatment is required. This can be either conventional or homoeopathic. Always ensure a well-balanced diet, which is high in iron content.

Remedies to consider:

Carbo veg Recommended when the periods are profuse and early, with indigestion problems, especially gassy flatulence and fullness.

Dulcamara The periods are weak, often missed, especially after exposure to cold or damp.

Ferrum met The loss is initially intermittent, or early and heavy. There may be weakness with shortness of breath on effort and anaemia.

Graphites For slight, or delayed periods, with pain and often constipation.

Magnesium carb The period is late, with a thick dark scanty loss. Exhaustion and sensitivity to noise is a feature.

Natrum mur The flow is irregular and unpredictable, often heavy, and associated with mood changes.

Platina The periods are early, also heavy, with clots and cramping pains. Irritability and arrogance are characteristic features.

Sepia The loss is heavy with clots, a severe dragging down pelvic discomfort and mood irritability.

PERIOD PROBLEMS

ABSENT

The periods are often delayed in adolescence, the age of onset of the first period, varying between ten and seventeen years, with an average of eleven or twelve. If the periods have not been established by the age of seventeen then professional advice should be sought. The periods may have never started, or after a few menstrual cycles, stopped for a period of months. Treatment always depends on the overall physical maturity of the teenager. Usually breast development and pubic hair is normal. But if there are any symptoms of physical immaturity, the breasts small or underdeveloped, or pubic hair absent or scanty, this may require a homoeopathic constitutional treatment, before the problem can be fully corrected.

If the mother or grandmother were late starting their menstrual cycle, then the cause may be an inherited one and the delay is without significance.
Other causes of delayed onset, are due to an endocrine (hormone producing glands) abnormality, for example adrenal or thyroid malfunctioning. Anorexia nervosa is another cause, the normal female cycle is not established due to the excessive weight loss and understimulation of the ovaries. A severe emotional shock or trauma may also affect the onset of menstruation, although it does not usually have a permanent effect on the cycle. More rarely the problem occurs after a physical illness which weakens the young teenager at this critical time in her development and causes delay.

Remedies to consider:

Aconitum   When this is due to an acute emotional shock or fright.

Belladonna   There is a feeling of burning warmth and restlessness, sometimes fear and anxiety.

Bryonia   The cause is often excessive movement, as from prolonged car, plane, or bus journeys.

Calcarea   Weakness occurs, with sweating and loss of confidence. The cause may be exposure to cold or damp.

Ignatia   The cause is an acute grief reaction with severe depression.

Kali carb   The commencement of the periods is delayed, the teenager anxious, over-weight and lacking energy and drive.

Pulsatilla   For the shy anxious teenager with variable periods, over-emotional and lacking confidence. Tears and sudden mood changes are common.

Sepia   The problem is associated with dragging down colicky pains, exhaustion and irritability.

PERIOD PROBLEMS

SPOTTING

Spotting, or slight breakthrough bleeding, is common for many adolescents, occurring in the mid-cycle at the time of ovulation. The cause is rupture of a few follicle cells on the surface of the ovary, with slight bleeding from minute blood vessels. It usually does not require any specific treatment unless severe, painful, or it has become a problem.

'Spotting' is often associated with using the contraceptive 'pill' and if the one you are taking does not suit you or regularly causes this type of problem it usually needs changing to a different type.

Other common causes of mid-cycle loss are:- bleeding after intercourse (often helped by using a lubricant and ensuring that intercourse is not rushed, the position chosen is completely comfortable), bleeding from a cervical polyp or erosion, or loss of blood because of an early spontaneous miscarriage. When due to miscarriage, there is usually a dark loss which is an isolated occurrence and associated with lower abdominal cramping pains.

Remedies to consider:

China   The problem is associated with exhaustion and intermittent fever, with a mild temperature. There is intolerance of draughts of cold air and touch.

Nitric acid   The problem is associated with stitch-like or splinter pelvic pains which are better for movement and aggravated by heat.

Pulsatilla   The remedy for great variability of symptoms, with everything unpredictable. All symptoms are aggravated by heat and an absence of fresh air. There are always surging dramatic emotions, especially floods of tears.

PREMENSTRUAL TENSION

Premenstrual tension or PMT is usually not severe during the adolescent years, but it can occur in a mild form. The causes of PMT are not fully understood, but usually considered to be due to hormonal imbalance, with high levels of oestrogen (the hormone produced in the first part of the female cycle), and low levels of progesterone (produced in the second half of the cycle). A few cases (5%), are due to high levels of prolactin (the hormone responsible for lactation).

The main symptoms teenagers experience are:- pre-period headache, fatigue, swollen or aching joints and a tendency to becoming accident-prone or clumsy. Before their period, most girls are much more emotional and vulnerable as feelings come to the surface. There may be floods of tears, impatience, irritability or short-fuse anger.

Most of the symptoms are due to fluid retention, because of an altered sodium/potassium balance, and high oestrogen levels. The mood changes are believed to be due to fluid retention within the nervous system, particularly at a cerebral (brain) level. The increased body fluid causes tender often painful breasts, or swelling of the fingers and ankles. The condition usually improves immediately the flow starts and does not recur until about a week before the next period.

Remedies to consider:

Ammonium carb Irritability, worse during stormy conditions, the periods heavy and too frequent.

Belladonna There is restless anxiety with increased aggressive behaviour, the periods heavy and often early.

Causticum The teenager is usually very sympathetic and sensitive, becoming depressed before the cycle, which is irregular. All symptoms are better for lying down at night.

Kali carb Anxiety with lack of energy is marked, the flow often heavy and late.

Natrum mur There is overwhelming anxiety, often with depression as the cycle begins. The periods tend to be irregular and are usually very heavy.

Nux vomica Spasms of pain during the cycle, associated with severe irritability and constipation.

Sepia There is a dragging-down pelvic discomfort, with irritability and fatigue, better for exercise and before thunder.

PSORIASIS

A chronic skin condition of unknown cause, which is not hereditary or infective. Psoriasis is usually mild in adolescence, causing scattered, dry, raised, circular or irregular areas of itchy skin redness, with thickening and sometimes severe flaking, which may crack or bleed.

The psoriasis thickening can occur on any part of the skin, but it is most common on exposed areas - particularly the elbows, knees, forehead, and scalp.It is also seen on the thighs, legs, arms and hands, back, abdomen, ears, under the nails and the genital area.

Psoriasis is often temporarily improved by a holiday, also from exposure to sunlight, sea air and sea bathing, but especially helped by rest and lowered stress levels. It tends to recur in a busy or pressurised home or work environment. If chronic and severe, psoriasis may also involve the joints, with stiffness and discomfort.

In some adolescents, the underlying temperament tends towards perfection with unreasonably high levels of expectation and targets of attainment. Intolerance, self-criticism with fear of failure is often present, making life a constant demand and a pressure. As a result the young teenager feels anxious, exhausted and vulnerable, under constant self-induced tension. Where there is a high level of emotional strain, psoriasis acts as an outlet for the emotional pressures engendered.

Psoriasis responds well to homoeopathy, a more balanced diet and reducing stress levels.

Remedies to consider:

Arsenicum   The skin itches and burns, red and swollen, often worse at night after midnight and aggravated by cold air and better for warm applications.

Borax   This remedy is useful for psoriasis of the scalp, aggravated by heat and better for cool air or cold applications.

Graphites   The psoriasis oozes a clear or straw-coloured discharge, the condition aggravated by heat and at night.

Petroleum   For dry, thick and crusty eruptions, which crack and bleed easily, aggravated by damp humid conditions and for cold.

Psorinum   The area affected is dry, grey or dirty-looking and very irritating. All symptoms are worse for heat or barometric changes.

Sulphur   For chronic problems which tend to become infected, crack, ooze, and bleed. All symptoms are worse for heat and for contact with water.

PUBERTY, DELAYED

The normal secondary sexual characteristics may fail to develop at the expected time. In the male these are the development of the pubic and body hair, erections, growth in size of the penis. For the female the important signs of puberty are the development of pubic hair, breast growth and changes and the onset of the menstrual cycle. In both sexes there is usually evidence of these changes beginning to occur over a period of one to two years before the full onset of puberty.

Delay may be due to hereditary causes where the mother or father also had a late onset, or they may be caused by hormonal imbalance. Other common reasons for puberty delay are:- severe and sustained stress, constant travelling or crisis movement, as may occur in a conflict situation. Delay may also occur from severe nutritional deficiency.

Because of television and the media, most teenagers are now fully aware of their approaching puberty and concerned when it will occur. They will usually discuss the onset of puberty with friends at school and more or less overtly, compare body shape and development, to assess their progress. Because it is a matter of such priority at this age, physical development should be noted by the parents and any delay, discussed with the adolescent and your doctor. In this way, if treatment is required, it can be started without delay, the teenager reassured, to keep stress, and anxiety minimal.

Remedies to consider:

Baryta carb   For the small immature teenager, with previous delays in all his developmental milestones.

Calcarea   The teenager is overweight and slow, with offensive sweats of the body, head and scalp, delayed in his development milestones and always cold.

Sabal serrulata   A useful remedy for delayed sexual maturation and lack of energy. Sympathy and concern gives rise to irritability.

Tuberculinum   A remedy for long-standing problems of the thin, tall adolescent who is sensitive to a chill or cold air and likes to be constantly on the move and travelling. Energy is either very low or quickly expended.

SEXUAL ANXIETY

This is an increasing problem, as teenagers are having sexual intercourse at an earlier age than in the past and although physically mature, they are emotionally immature. In the US, many teenagers aged eleven or twelve experience their first sexual relationships, and by the mid-teens, 30% of girls and 60% of boys are sexually active. The figures are comparable in the UK, and there is an increasing risk of AIDS from unprotected heterosexual intercourse. In the three years 1988-1991, AIDS affected 0.4 to 1.8% of the US teenage population.

Sexual anxieties occur because of emotional immaturity, with typical teenage pressures to perform, respond, conform to his peer-group expected 'norm' and causing a wide variety of problems and difficulties. These include general emotional upsets, especially depression and anxiety. There may be more specific problems, including frigidity, anxiety about achieving orgasm, vaginismus (vaginal spasm during intercourse), premature ejaculation and various potency problems.
The problems are made worse because they cause fear or shame and because they cannot be easily talked about to parents or friends.

Sexuality is often thrust upon a young teenager, who although mature physically, is not sure of himself or confident, able to communicate fully and to relate at a mature level. Problems should be talked through and understood at the time, ideally within the teenage couple relationship, or with a close friend, or trusted member of the family.

Remedies to consider:

Argentum nit   Where fear and obsessional anxiety is predominant. There is intolerance of heat.

Ignatia   Indicated where a sexual problem is linked to unresolved problems of grief, loss, or separation anxiety.

Lycopodium   A remedy for the anxious immature teenager who appears more in control of his emotions than he is in reality. Anticipatory anxiety is usually the major problem area.

Pulsatilla   Recommended for the bashful shy adolescent, often an only child with little social experience with the opposite sex. Mood changes and shifts of feeling cause relationship difficulties. Tearful depression is characteristic and there is usually intolerance of heat.

Sulphur   A remedy for recurrent severe problems, avoiding sharing, closeness, and emotional commitment. There is an excessive preoccupation with vague plans and ideas.

SHYNESS

This is always an uncomfortable, often painful, psychological state for any teenager. There is a strong wish to withdraw into the background, yet at the same time, paradoxically there is also a need to be noticed and for attention. In many ways, this is a fundamental dilemma for the shy adolescent, who often fails to realise, that at the same time as seeking withdrawal and retreating from others, he is also seeking to place himself in the limelight.

Much of the root cause of shyness is based in misplaced sexual anxiety and guilt, which the adolescent feels unable to talk about or to express. The biological libidinal drive, is felt to be bad and wrong and their clear healthy interest in sexual attraction and relationships has therefore to be expressed indirectly through painful shyness, rather than in a more open and direct way.

The shy teenager does not accept himself as a complex young adult, with a wide variety of needs, feelings and expressions. He tends to feel everything in extremes, either bad, guilt-ridden, or a failure. The problem occurs because he is never at ease with himself and this is what is experiences with others outside his immediate peer group, especially in a mixed group. The shy adolescent is often an only child, or effectively so, because his siblings are much older or younger. This may leave him with little opportunity to play and socialise with them and to gain experience of the opposite sex at an early age. Shyness is best dealt with by a very varied family social life and free and open discussion of all emotional and sexual topics.

Remedies to consider:

Arsenicum   For the teenager who is a loner, avoiding others, often excessively neat and tidy. Depressive moods.

Gelsemium   For milder problems, in an insecure dramatic adolescent who needs constant reassurance. There is a tendency to withdraw.

Lycopodium   For the pseudo-mature adolescent who appears older than his years, because he is more at ease with older or younger age-groups, but tends to avoid his own peer group.

Natrum mur   For the anxious, often depressed and more deeply psychologically disturbed adolescent, who lacks confidence in every social situation and can never ever be really himself with others.

Pulsatilla   A major remedy for shyness problems in either the male or female adolescent, with a constant need to gain attention, yet at the same time he is terrified by the limelight. Bashful shyness can be severe, although it is also variable. Aggression is usually either denied, or directed at the self by self-critical tendencies.

119

SORE THROAT

This is usually of infective origin and part of either an acute cold or viral flu epidemic. It can also be associated with allergy or trauma to the area. Symptoms occur because of invasion of the tonsil or back of the throat with an acute viral or bacterial organism, causing pain and swelling of the area, frequently with a raised temperature.

The main symptoms are pain or discomfort on swallowing or talking, the glands in the neck swollen and tender. There may be loss of appetite, lack of energy and a general feeling of malaise, sometimes with a high temperature. Pain may spread to one or both ears, or involve the sinuses, causing headache, or nasal catarrh. Usually the problem is short-lived and clears completely within a few days. If a sore throat persists, (especially if you are taking a prescribed medication), always consult your doctor to ensure that a throat infection is not due to the side-effects of any medication you are taking.

Most adolescents recover quickly from a sore throat with homoeopathy. This should however always be combined with commonsense precautions - keeping warm, rest, plenty of hot drinks with lemon and honey and a light easily digestible diet until the sore throat has completely cleared.

If a teenager has a high temperature, he can still use homoeopathy, but if it persists, he should have a medical opinion. Bed rest and plenty of fluids, is essential until the temperature is normal.

Remedies to consider:

Aconitum
For acute throat infections, the area hot, dry, red and swollen. The throat feels narrowed and swallowing is uncomfortable.

Baryta carb
There is an acutely inflamed throat, with stitch-like pain in the area. The lymphatic glands in the neck and under the jaw may be tender and enlarged. Swallowing of solids is painful.

Belladonna
For acute inflammation, with a raised temperature. The throat is red and feels dry.

Hepar sulph
There is an acute throat condition with stitch-like pains on movement and swallowing. Irritability is marked.

Kali carb
For left-sided acute throat infections. The area feels rough, dry and sore. Swallowing is difficult. All symptoms are worse in the early night hours.

Lachesis
A remedy for acute left-sided conditions. The throat is a deep purple colour and may bleed.

Mercurius
For right-sided conditions with a high temperature and sweating.

STEALING

Theft is one of the most common social problems in our society. It varies from petty theft - a purse or wallet taken from home or school - to more severe forms, including theft of cars and breaking-in to property. When stealing is a localised problem, only occurring within the immediate family unit, it nearly always reflects an emotional disturbance of some kind, either mild and transitory. There may be a more profound psychological disturbance if the acts are repeated over a period.

Often the adolescent is insecure or jealous, and feels pushed-out by another sibling or new parental partner who has moved in. He may believe that the new member of the family is more loved, wanted or valued, the stealing a symbolic way of retrieving the love, admiration, status or attention he feels is now denied him. It may also express a revenge motive, the anger, deprivation and anger he feels, but is unable to express.

Where stealing is more of a social group problem, it often reflects a break-down of family values and closeness, lack of supervision, absent or very impoverished communication, often an environment that is deprived of parks or leisure facilities. It is especially associated with high rise blocks, unemployment, poverty, noise, pollution and overcrowding. Stealing may also reflect social depression, in an area where families feel denied, forgotten, or undervalued, with little sense of worth or hope for the future. In these situations, stealing is as an expression of anger, an outlet for the basic human need to fill an inner psychological vacuum.

Remedies to consider:

Ignatia
The problem is related to unresolved grief and loss, a manifestation of underlying depression.

Natrum mur
For the teenager with severe psychological problems of depression or anxiety. Stealing may be an attempt to attract attention and help for his problems, or to take flight from them. Theft gives a temporary high if successful, but eventually it fails to satisfy or push away the real problem area and depression returns, often more severely.

Nux vomica
A remedy to consider for the angry, often irritable teenager, who feels misunderstood, abandoned or rejected by the world - usually meaning his family. He may steal deliberately to symbolically pay back society (representing the parental figures), or to denigrate them by the acts of theft.

Platina
For the rather arrogant teenager who steals to show his superiority, but beneath the surface feels depressed and inadequate.

STOMACH CRAMPS

These often occur in adolescents, due either to hunger when a meal has been missed, or because of acute indigestion, particularly when food has been eaten too quickly. A burger or pizza, eaten standing up, in a fast-food take-away, still needs to be chewed, each mouthful thoroughly masticated and broken down, so that digestion can occur.

Some of the other causes are: - smoking, which diminishes appetite, so that food is eaten as a habit, rather than savoured with relish and enjoyment. Drinking excessive amounts of alcohol, tea, or coffee, which are acidic, irritates the lining layer of the stomach, causing congestion and thickening, with loss of appetite, nausea, and cramping discomfort.

Another common cause of stomach cramps is eating food of poor quality - either too sweet or spicy, or containing a very high animal fat content. Eating infected food may also cause gastritis (inflammation of the stomach wall).

If pain and cramps are recurrent, with severe discomfort occurring immediately or a few hours after eating, the adolescent may have a stomach or duodenal ulcer which requires specialised treatment over a periods of several weeks or longer.

Note that stress in any form, has an immediate effect on the normal process of digestion within the stomach and may cause nausea, indigestion, loss of appetite, or stomach cramps.

Remedies to consider:

Chelidonium For right-sided pains, the tongue yellow, with vomiting or nausea, a bitter taste in the mouth and marked lethargy or exhaustion. All symptoms are worse for movement or touch.

Magnesium phos A remedy for severe colicky pains with flatulence and distention of the upper abdominal region. Belching is a feature but gives little relief from the pain which is however helped by local heat, as from a hot water bottle.

Nux vomica This remedy is recommended for spasms of upper pain with nausea or vomiting and marked irritability. Symptoms are relieved by firm local pressure and humid moist conditions.

Pulsatilla For variable indigestion pains, often caused by dietary excess from either a rich fatty meal or too many carbohydrates. There is great intolerance of heat in any form and thirst is absent. Varying dramatic emotional moods are characteristic.

SWEATING

Teenage sweating is an unpleasant worrying problem, which may be caused by several factors. Any form of infection, with a raised body temperature causes sweating to occur in an attempt to cool the body by the surface evaporation of moisture. Other common causes are:- exhaustion and weakness, lack of resistance and impaired vitality. Sweating is also associated with the lack of drive and energy which occurs in post-viral M.E. syndromes, with profound exhaustion, muscular pains and weakness. It is also common when a teenager is tired, or in any way under par.

Sweating may occur after a long drawn-out debilitating illness - influenza, glandular fever, and when convalescing - perhaps after surgery, following viral pneumonia or a more severe infection, as meningitis, pyelitis (inflammation of the kidney) also after adolescent mumps.

Stress and emotional factors are other causes of outbreaks of sweating, particularly when the teenager feels under pressure, ill-at-ease or vulnerable and that he is not coping well. Sweating is a frequent symptom of problems of insecurity, guilt, or shyness. Whenever sweating occurs which is of emotional origin, it is helpful if the parents try to clarify the underlying reasons and are positive in their support. Teenagers should be encouraged to talk about sexuality and their personal problems, in a simple direct way.

Remedies to consider:

Ipecacuanha   A remedy where sweating is associated with severe and persistent nausea or vomiting. All symptoms are aggravated by lying down and warm stuffy conditions.

Pulsatilla   Indicated when associated with emotional tension, shyness and anxiety. The symptoms are typically variable, aggravated by heat, crowds and new social situations.

Pyrogen   For sweating linked to a raised temperature and an acute infection.

Thuja   The sweating is offensive, the adolescent dark-complexioned. Multiple warts occur and fatigue the least effort. Sweating is worse from any form of heat, in the early night hours from 3-4.00 am, from eating fats and from coffee.

TONSILLITIS

Acute inflammation of the tonsils is one of the commonest causes of an acute sore throat in adolescence. It may be of viral or bacterial origin, with or without a raised temperature. In most cases the throat is sore, red and tender, usually very painful on swallowing, with enlarged tender lymph glands in the neck area. Ear-ache may also occur because of a secondary infection from the throat area.

Tonsillitis is often an acute sudden illness, which follows a cold and lasts for a week to ten days before the throat feels normal again. But it can also be a recurrent problem, especially when the resistance of the teenager is low and he is constantly exposed to colds and throat infections at college or university.

If tonsillitis becomes a chronic or recurrent problem, never really clearing up completely, so that every few weeks there is a recurrence of a painful throat, it may drag the teenager down, as the infection undermines health, drive, energy and vitality. When this happens, a constitutional prescription is often indicated, best prescribed by your homoeopathic doctor.

Remedies to consider:

Baryta carb   For acute problems, the tonsils enlarged, with sharp, stitching pain on swallowing. The throat is dark red or purple, with, relief from fresh cool air.

Belladonna   A remedy for very acute tonsillitis, the area bright red, dry and glazed looking. There is a raised temperature and swallowing is usually painful.

Calcium phos   There is severe swelling of the tonsillar region, causing pain and great difficulty in swallowing.

Hepar sulph   There are sharp stitch or splinter-like pains around the tonsil, worse for swallowing solids. The throat is red and dry, the temperature raised. Irritability is a marked feature.

Lachesis   For left-sided tonsillitis, the area dark red or purple plum coloured. There is extreme tenderness, the pain intensified by swallowing or the least pressure.

Mercurius   For right-sided infections which discharge a foul yellow pus. The temperature is raised, with sweating, apathy and exhaustion.

129

TRAVEL SICKNESS

Motion sickness is always an unpleasant distressing complaint. It is caused by an inner ear disturbance, due to the particular form of movement which affects the balance centres. It is common in children and teenagers and may be associated with sea, land, or air travel.

The exact mechanism is still not fully understood, but as well as disturbance of the balance centres, emotional factors also play an important role in the condition. Apprehension and any anticipation of the problem, tends to aggravate the condition in addition to other factors as vibration, judder, and stong fumes or odours (for example hot cooking oil or diesel fumes).

The condition is sometimes present in the most seasoned sailor, even after many years at sea and it can also occur in cross channel swimmers who suffer severe nausea from the buffeting rocking movements of waves.

Lying down, relaxing, resting quietly usually improves the nausea. The problem responds well to the homoeopathic approach which can also help with prevention.

Remedies to consider:

Borax The least downwards motion causes nausea and vomiting. The problem is also aggravated by heat and cigarette smoke.

Cocculus Dizziness with nausea is characteristic of this remedy, worse for all movement and for sitting up, The nauseais relieved by lying down.

Kreosotum There is nausea or vomiting, which is relieved by warmth and eating.

Nux vomica Nausea with irritability, improved by lying down and from sleeping.

Petroleum Nausea with the production of much clear watery mucus, relieved by eating.

Tabacum There is nausea with dizziness, worse from the smell of cigarettes. The pit of the stomach feels sinking and hollow. All symptoms are better for fresh air and worse from heat or cold air.

TRUANCY

This is a common teenage problem (about 3,000 a year in the UK, of which 500 are persistent, and may drift into juvenile crime). It often follows a similar pattern in childhood. Flight, or running away, is usually from school, but it may also be from the home, especially if the teenager feels unwanted, or the home environment is hostile and indifferent.

Truancy may be caused by bullying at school, either by other children, or sometimes by a teacher. The adolescent may feel unable to keep up with his school and homework demands, feeling inadequate and a failure, alienated from the other pupils, with few friends. He may see no future, either at home or in school, wanting to take his chance alone in one of the cities, often with other similar teenagers he has met. Drugs may become involved, or alcohol. There may also be the attraction of crime and easy money.

Many teenagers who truant, also experience a failure of communication in the home, the adolescent often feeling depressed, unloved, and unwanted. Usually he also feels misunderstood and that whatever he says will be cast into a critical mould, where his opinions and ideas will be seen as either, negative or unrealistic. He is often lonely and frequently undernourished. The problem usually begins in a minor way, as a warning symptom and at this stage it can be more easily treated and discussed within the family. Where truancy is deeply entrenched, it is more difficult to deal with because the adolescent may not be living with the parents or refuse to discuss his feelings and viewpoints. Counselling is often helpful.

Remedies to consider:

Aconitum
The underlying problem is fear and anxiety, e.g. a strong conviction that disaster is imminent for a sibling or parent to whom he has strong ambivalent feelings.

Gelsemium
Useful for mild problems where there is underlying insecurity and fear.

Lycopodium
A remedy for the apprehensive teenager who sees any change - in the home or at school, as a potential disaster, leading to flight and self-destructive behaviour.

Natrum mur
This remedy is of value where there is rigidity of attitudes, in a teenager who has few social contacts of his own age.

Nux vomica
For the difficult angry unhappy adolescent, who feels 'hard done by', convinced that his viewpoint is the right one. Irritability with depression and frustration.

Silicea
A remedy to consider for the weak, anxious teenager who lacks staying power in competitive situations and needing constant reassurance.

WARTS

Warts are usually firm localised swellings, which form on any part of the body. They occur on most people at some time and are caused by a viral infection of the area affected.

They vary considerably in shape and appearance and may be flat and small, or larger with a fleshy root to them and a head like a small cauliflower. They are particularly common on the fingers, but may occur on the face, chest, or feet.

Genital or anal warts, are a separate problem from those occurring elsewhere and are often associated with an underlying genital infection. If they persist, after homoeopathic treatment, they should be treated in a clinic which specialises in sexual problems.

Unless they are large, or causing pain, it is usually not wise to remove them and they are best left alone. Most warts shrivel up and disappear with homoeopathic treatment as the underlying health and resistance improves. A constitutional remedy may be if they are widespread or recurrent.

Remedies to consider:

Antimonium crud   For multiple warts, with mood irritability and digestive problems, such as loss of appetite. The tongue has a thick white coating. There is great intolerance of heat or sunlight.

Causticum   The warts are typically large, rough-looking and friable. They are often present on the finger tips or nose. Bleeding may occur.

Chelidonium   For chronic warts associated with apathy and exhaustion. There is a yellow discolouration of the tongue.

Dulcamara   The warts are smooth and large, particularly common on the hands and feet.

Nitric acid   For large irregular warts which bleed after washing.

Staphysagria   A remedy for single or multiple warts, often large and with a marked stem or peduncle.

Thuja   For chronic wart problems. The skin is pale, grey, and oily.

X-RAYS

Any form of x-ray investigation should be questioned as to its necessity and treated cautiously because they have an accumulative effect. All x-rays are potentially carcinogenic (cancer forming).

It is now standard medical policy to keep any form of x-ray exposure to a minimum and only to recommend them when strictly indicated. In the past, regular mass screening of the population, for the early diagnosis of lung disease was advocated. But this has now changed, and is no longer recommended, because the potential risks of frequent x-ray exposure, may be greater than the chest disease.

It is particularly important throughout pregnancy to avoid any form of x-ray exposure to the pregnant uterus, unless it is life-saving for the mother. This is true for all forms of x-rays, including dental or chiropractic films. Where a woman of child-bearing age, who is having intercourse, has a delayed period, she should assume that she may be pregnant and avoid any x-ray exposure to the young and very vulnerable early foetus, until the next cycle has begun. Where a patient has never felt well since exposure to x-rays, then homoeopathy may be of positive help.

Remedies to consider:

Radium brom   For the ill-effects of long-term
                      radiation exposure.

Thuja   Where the teenager has never
                      been well since exposure to
                      x-rays, with vague general malaise
                      and ill health. He may also
                      experience tearing pains in the
                      neck, scalp, muscles and joint
                      areas. All symptoms are worse for
                      chill or damp weather. Extremes
                      of exhaustion tend to occur from
                      the least effort.

X-Ray   The homoeopathic potency.

INDEX

OTHER INSIGHT PUBLICATIONS

HOMOEOPATHY

Understanding Homoeopathy

The revised second edition of this comprehensive book explains in clear, simple terms the basic principles of homoeopathy, which can be readily understood by the beginner. The author outlines the approach, indications, and choice of remedies for the common health problems of the family.

Talking About Homoeopathy

An invaluable reference book for anyone wishing to understand homoeopathy. The book covers a variety of topics of general interest which offer a deeper understanding and a more challenging awareness of homoeopathy, its indications, potential and scope of action.

The Principles, Art and Practice of Homoeopathy

A book which explains in simple language the principles of homoeopathic practice and prescribing. It includes chapters on :- Dosage, Potency, First and Second Prescriptions, Homoeopathic History Taking and The Consultation. A second section is concerned with Constitutional Prescribing, and the role of homoeopathy in the treatment of Cancer.

PSYCHOLOGY

Emotional Health

A unique and major study of the most common emotional problems facing society in the twentieth century. It identifies their causes and symptoms, and then explains the best, practical, self-help steps that can be taken to solve them. Simple guidelines are given in order to promote healthier attitudes, changes in specific problem areas, and better psychological perspectives.

Personal Growth and Creativity

A guide to the most effective ways to stimulate and develop personal creativity in order to bring about positive change in creative outlook. The book offers practical guidelines that will lead to constructive results.

RISKS OF MODERN LIVING

The Side-Effects Book

This books describes in detail the most common hazards of our pressurised society, the props used and their risk to health. Chapters include: Developmental Stages of life, Stress and the Home, Sexuality, Over-The-Counter Drugs, Health Products and Vitamins, Medically Prescribed Drugs, Surgical and Cosmetic Procedures, Immunisation, Food and Diet, Social Addictions, Holidays and the Sun, Travel, Sport, Occupations, Animals and Plants, Household Products, Pesticides, Drugs of Dependence and Misuse, Pollution.

Please send s.a.e. for a list of other health titles.